Healing
Root Causes and Solutions

A STEP-BY-STEP INTESTINAL REGENERATION PROGRAM

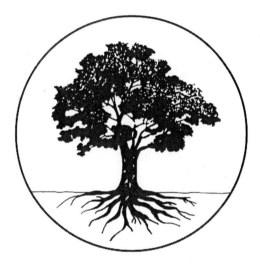

Food is the soil from which the tree
of our own life is grown.

Russell Mariani
Health Educator, Nutrition Counselor

Assisting in the quest for better health through better nutrition since 1980.

Specializing in the prevention and correction of digestive system imbalances.

All rights reserved. No part of this book may be reproduced or transmitted in any form or by any means, without the prior written permission of the author.

The information and suggestions contained in this book are based upon the research and experiences of the author, both personally and professionally. However, the information and suggestions in this book are not intended as a substitute for effective consultation with the health care professional of your choice. The publisher and author are not responsible for any adverse effects or consequences from the use of any suggestions, preparations, or procedures discussed in this book. All matters relevant to your physical health and well-being should be supervised by a caring and attentive health care professional. It is a sign of intelligence and enlightened self-interest to seek a second or third opinion about your condition and symptoms and how you can become more proactive in your own self care.

Second Edition
Published by: Maramor Press
Editor: Lentmerch Orfolding
Copy Editor: Rosie Pearson
Proofreader: Nina Perry
Illustrations: Teri Susmita Wikinson
The Great American Pastime, page 63 & 227; Sue Dewar
Production, book and cover design: Robert B. Smyth
Cover Photo: Kevin Ebi - Used with permission
Back Cover Photo: Michael J. Charles Photography - Used with permission

Permissions: *Some Essential Information About Salt*, article used by permission; The Grain & Salt Society; *Faith is a Magic* used by permission; Odds Bodkin. Every effort has been made to obtain permission to reprint all pieces. If necessary the proper credit will be added in all future editions.

Special Thanks to Jim Parker and Paul Fitzgerald

Copyright 2006 & 2014 by Russell Mariani
ISBN: 0-9786703-0-2 - 1st Edition
ISBN: 978-0-9786703-3-7 - 2nd Edition

Library of Congress Cataloging-in-Publication Data
Mariani, Russell, 1955–
Healing Digestive Illness; Root Causes and Solutions
A Step-By-Step Intestinal Regeneration Program

For information about upcoming lectures, seminars, retreats, on-line classes and individual consultations please visit Russell's web site:
www.healingdigestiveillness.com

Maramor Press
514 Amherst Road
South Hadley, MA 01075
(413) 536 - 3322

DEDICATION

This book is dedicated to the imminent achievement of one peaceful world through the biological transformation of humanity. The biological transformation of humanity will be achieved through a deeper understanding of and a vigorous commitment to all aspects of what we could call a *comprehensive ecological literacy*. This literacy would include, but not be limited to the following things: respect for our ancestors, each other, and all living things; nourishing habits based upon nourishing traditions; and wiser choices about everything based upon common sense.

Be Well
Russell Mariani

Table Of Contents

Author's Note to the Reader

SECTION ONE
GETTING READY

Welcome! --2
The Purpose of This Book ---3
There Are Three Kinds of Knowledge -----------------------------5
Russell's Rules for Optimal Digestion ----------------------------8
Do You Know Anyone with Digestive System Problems? ------- 10
Why I Am Writing This Book ----------------------------------- 13
The Most Common Digestive System Problems ---------------- 16
What Is "The Cause" of All These Problems? ------------------- 19
Root Cause #1 - Chronic Unintentional Dehydration ------------ 20
Root Cause #2 - Nutritional Deficiencies --------------------------- 24
Root Cause #3 - Nutritional Excess ------------------------------- 28
Root Cause #4 - Intestinal Dysbiosis ----------------------------- 29
Root Cause #5 - Stress --- 31
Is There a "Cure" For All These Problems? --------------------- 33
What Is Functional Nutrition? ----------------------------------- 36
Biological Principle Number One: Homeostasis ----------------- 40
Complementary Habit Number One: Be Proactive! ------------ 42
Functional Nutrition and the Period of Adjustment -------------- 44
Giving Thanks for Our Food ------------------------------------ 46
A Quick Tour through the Digestive System ------------------- 47
The Ideal Bowel Movement ------------------------------------- 58
Checking Our Transit Time ------------------------------------- 60
The Power of True Stories -------------------------------------- 64
Russell's Story: Ulcerative Colitis, Anxiety, Depression ---------- 69

Grant's Story: Ulcerative Colitis ------------------------------------ 82
Brittany's Story: Extreme Constipation --------------------------- 86
Mike's Story: Crohn's Disease ----------------------------------- 88
Maxine's Story: Acute Diverticulitis ---------------------------- 94
Bob's Story: IBS, Acid Reflux, and Much More!------------------ 95
Jessica's Story: Extreme Gas and Bloating ---------------------- 98
Your Story: Five Vital Question Areas   ------------------------ 100

SECTION TWO
GETTING STARTED

Introduction to Section Two ----------------------------------- 105
The Healing Power of Commitment ------------------------------- 108
The Key Problem Areas (A Quick Review)-------------------------- 110
Three Types of Bowel Movement Problems ------------------------- 113
The Three Phases of Your Intestinal Regeneration Program ------ 115
Phase One: What to Do Next ------------------------------------- 118
Exercise Mindfulness --- 119
The Watercure Recipe --- 120
Why Is Proper Daily Hydration So Important? ------------------- 128
Purchasing Your Celtic Sea Salt from
The Grain and Salt Society ------------------------------------- 130
Supplements to Order --- 131
How to Use the Supplements ------------------------------------- 133
Specific Product Usage Guidelines ------------------------------ 134
Your New Food Program: Phase One Foods Simplified -------- 141
What to eat? --- 144
Your Old and New Breakfast Routine ----------------------------- 145
Whole Grain Porridge: Basic Cooking Instructions -------------- 149
What About Lunch and Dinner? ----------------------------------- 151
Basic Miso Soup -- 153
Tamari Tea: Quick Remedy for Gas and Bloating --------------- 155
Please Read This Paragraph Before Moving On
(Or Giving Up!)--- 156
The Habits of Functional Nutrition ----------------------------- 157
Complementary or Insulting? ----------------------------------- 163
Practice These Complementary Habits Consistently! ----------- 164
Avoid These Insulting Habits as Much as Possible! -------------- 167
The Seven Day Experiment -------------------------------------- 170
The Power of Choice: Your Key To a Successful Phase One --- 172
The Power of Our Core Beliefs----------------------------------- 174
The Road Not Taken --- 178

SECTION THREE
OPTIMIZING RESULTS

The Purpose of Section Three --------------------------------- 181
The Modern Cornucopia --- 182
The Truth About Whole Grains ---------------------------------- 187
Toxicology and Human Health ----------------------------------- 189
What are toxic and hazardous chemicals? ----------------------- 190
How to Find Certified Organic Foods --------------------------- 194
Each Cell Is a Factory -- 195
According to Our Factory Metaphor
How Do We Stay Healthy? --------------------------------------- 197
Phase One Foods --- 199
Reflective Practice --- 201
Some Essential Information About Salt ------------------------- 203
The Negative Impacts of Cold Foods and Beverages -------------- 206
Some Thoughts on Acid and Alkaline Food Balances -------------- 208
Why Use Supplemental Digestive Enzymes? ----------------------- 212
Uses of Digestive Enzymes ------------------------------------- 214
Why Probiotic Supplements Are So Important -------------------- 217
What Do the Acidophilus Bacteria Do? -------------------------- 220
How to Expand Your Breakfast Menu ----------------------------- 228
What is Nutrigenomics? -- 231
My Favorite Recipes for Phase One ----------------------------- 233
The Conscious Breathing Exercise ------------------------------ 250
Therapeutic Abdominal Massage --------------------------------- 253
Eat Light and Eat Early --------------------------------------- 256
The Habits: Daily and Weekly Checklists ----------------------- 259

SECTION FOUR
WHAT'S NEXT?

About the Author -- 265
Resources --- 267
Sources for Organic Quality Whole Foods ----------------------- 271
Great Cookbooks, DVD's, & Cooking Instructors ----------------- 273
Residential Programs -- 274
Lab Testing --- 275
Select Bibliography --- 276
Acknowledgements -- 283
What Lies Ahead? -- 285
Faith is a Magic -- 287
The Last Word --- 288

LIST OF ILLUSTRATIONS

The Human Digestive System	48
Cross Section of the Small Intestine	54, 219
The Normal Colon	55, 223
The Abnormal Colon	56, 225
Length of Digestive System Comparison	59
The Great American Pastime	63, 227
Dis-eases of the Digestive System	111
Each Cell is a Factory	196

🌰 Author's Note to the Reader

I am not a medical doctor. The information in this book should not be used or thought of as medical advice. If you need medical advice for your condition please seek it out right away from the appropriate medical professionals. I work alongside my clients in cooperation with their medical doctors, including their gastroenterologists, internists, and surgeons. There are a growing number of medical doctors who are familiar with the information and approaches described in these pages in addressing digestive system problems. These medical doctors will encourage you to follow my guidelines and suggestions. Unfortunately these "Functional Medicine Doctors" are still few and far between, but you will meet some of them in these pages. Other medical doctors still maintain the position that "diet and lifestyle" are not the *root cause* of digestive system problems. Some of these medical doctors will discourage you from trying anything on your own, and not take the time to examine the relevancy and efficacy of the material in this book or other books. If this is your current situation you may want to seek out a second or third opinion. Still, other medical doctors will take the position that changing your diet is a good thing, but not necessarily *the* thing that is going to make a big difference in your condition. These doctors often say: "I don't see how improving your diet could harm you in any way, so go ahead; just don't expect it to improve your medical condition." We have a lot of work ahead of us to more fully integrate the many discoveries and re-discoveries in the area of diet and lifestyle into the world of allopathic medicine and our current health care system. Time will tell.

If you are not currently a client of mine, then I cannot possibly know all the details of your symptoms and condition. I cannot possibly know all the various circumstances that have led up to the choices you are making in your current diet and lifestyle. This fact should not prevent you from benefiting from the information and suggestions in this book. Just take your time, and use common sense. And please feel free to contact me directly for information about becoming a client.

My goal in this book is to provide information and suggestions which have been utilized successfully by thousands of other people in their own self-healing process. If I am not directly involved with you as your counselor and guide, I cannot guarantee your results. However, I can and will guarantee you this: that every word and suggestion in this book is totally dedicated and committed to optimizing your self-healing journey.

If you are ready to become more proactive in your own self-care, this is the book for you. If you are ready to "experiment" and take more complete personal responsibility for your own condition and your own results, then this book will be extremely helpful to you. If you are willing to read these pages with a grain of salt and determine what makes sense to you and what doesn't, this book will open new paths for your own self-healing journey. If you are willing to identify the things that nourish you best, and then consistently do the things that nourish you best, you will have learned the greatest lesson of all.

Russell Mariani

All you have to decide is what
to do with the time that is given to you.
Gandalf The Gray

Section One
GETTING READY

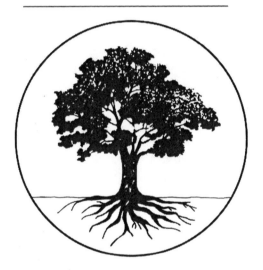

Food is the soil from which the tree of our own life is grown.

Section 1 - Getting Ready

Welcome!

Thank you for purchasing this book. You have just made an important investment in your own personal health and healing journey. This investment has the ability to pay you dividends every day for the rest of your life. Make a commitment *right now* to read each paragraph and every page and follow each suggestion with complete attention to every detail. You will not fail. You will succeed in taking the steps and making the changes that your digestive system requires of you; *so that your own digestive system inside your own body* will heal itself. Teaching people how to cooperate with the dynamic healing systems inside their own body is the essence of the work that I do. I have been doing this work since 1980. I am passionate about teaching others how to become more proactive in their own self-care. This book is a precise summary of the exact same program I use with my clients in my private practice. The testimonials you have already read, or will read about soon are all the result of people just like you following the program described in these pages. I did it. They did it. And so can you! Now, let's get started!

> *The doctor of the future will give no medicine,*
> *but will interest his patients in the care of the human frame,*
> *in diet, and in the cause and prevention of disease.*
> Thomas A. Edison

Section 1 - *Getting Ready*

🌰 *The Purpose of This Book*

The purpose of this book is to teach you how to heal yourself from your current digestive system problems, whatever they are, and no matter how long you have been suffering. Your ability to do this depends upon your learning the basic principles and practices of what I have come to call *Functional Nutrition*. Functional Nutrition refers to the dietary and lifestyle habits that; *when practiced consistently*, have the ability to restore normal physiological functioning to the cells, organs and systems of your body. Normal physiological functioning is the foundation for all physical health and the surest path to a life without dis-ease. Ultimately, Functional Nutrition is the answer to one very important question: *What nourishes me best?* That is to say: What nourishes *you* best!

The first phase of your *Intestinal Regeneration Program* will result in the relief from whatever troubling symptoms you are currently experiencing. The second phase will be to physically rebuild your digestive system: cell by cell, section by section until you are able to digest, absorb, assimilate, and eliminate a wide variety of foods and beverages with optimum comfort and ease. The third and final phase of your *Intestinal Regeneration Program* will find you experiencing a level of health and vitality you may never have experienced before. The best way to describe this level of health is: *the experience of total dietary freedom.*

I want you to be free to eat whatever you want to eat whenever you want to eat it.

Imagine that.

Any dietary or lifestyle *restrictions* that you may encounter during the first two phases of your *Intestinal Regeneration Program* are temporary. How temporary? Usually a few weeks to a few months time is all that is required. You need to learn how to restore normal functioning to your digestive system. In order to do that, you need to quiet things down, calm things down, and settle things down inside your digestive system. In order to do that, you need to select foods and beverages that complement normal intestinal functioning and you need to avoid (like the plague) any foods and beverages that may be insulting to normal intestinal functioning. Just remember that any food and beverage restrictions are temporary and necessary to restore normal functioning to your digestive system and you will do just fine, like the thousands of people who have come before you.

To me, the very best definition of health is this: *the ability to digest anything.*

Imagine that.

When you achieve the goal of *total dietary freedom* is completely up to you. My job is to teach you the most important fundamentals and provide you with a reliable map and compass for the journey ahead. Getting to the destination of *total dietary freedom* is an adventure unique to each of us, and no one else can take us *all the way there*. We make the way ourselves, one step at a time, one day at a time, one decision at a time.

I wish you well on your journey to total dietary health and freedom and I hope this book provides you with many clues about how to achieve such a wonderful, life-changing goal.

Section 1 - Getting Ready

🌰 *There Are Three Kinds of Knowledge*

What you *need* to know. What is *nice* to know. What is *nuts* to know. (That is, as it relates to your desire to get well as soon as possible.)

This book is filled with *need to know* information so that you can take the steps and make the necessary changes that will produce *intestinal regeneration* in your own body. As this happens, the digestive system problems you are currently suffering from will gradually and *sometimes rapidly* disappear. It will be totally up to you whether you invite them back to ruin your life again or not. Health is a choice. Your health is a direct result of all your choices but especially your choices about *what* to eat and drink; and when and where and how and why, as you are about to discover.

(Or re-discover!)

Your body wants to be healthy. Your body is genetically programmed to be healthy. Your body has the capacity to regenerate and heal and then remain healthy and disease-free, but to do so, it requires your conscious and consistent cooperation. The *need to know* information in this book will show you exactly how to cooperate with the dynamic self-healing mechanisms inside your own body; inside your own digestive system. There is no one single *magic bullet* that produces such fantastic results. Healing is the result of consistently making the choices that nourish and activate the amazing self-healing capacities waiting patiently inside every one of our 100 trillion-plus *cells*.

> Human beings originate from a single cell. This cell divides into two other cells, which in turn divide themselves and this division continues on indefinitely.

> In the course of this process of structural elaboration and construction, the embryo retains the functional simplicity of the original single-celled egg. The cells of the human body seem to remember their original unity, even when they have organized and become the elements of an innumerable multitude. Each cell understands spontaneously and intuitively the functions required of it inside the organized whole. This innate knowledge of the part they must play in the manifestation of a healthy, wholesome body, is a *consciousness* or mode of being inside each and every cell. (Alexis Carrel, *Man the Unknown* [London: Universe Books, 1961], 55)

Imagine that. Each cell in your body *understands spontaneously and intuitively the functions required of them inside the organized whole.* This is a more poetic way of saying that "your body is genetically programmed to be healthy" as I stated above. Of course this would include the cells that make up your digestive system too. *This innate knowledge of the part they must play in the manifestation of a healthy, wholesome body is a consciousness or mode of being inside each and every cell.* Imagine what this means in practical, everyday terms. If every cell in your body is so smart and so resourceful, doesn't it make sense to take better care of them? Start imagining what your life would be like if *the care of your cells* became the number one priority of your life.

Imagination is more important than knowledge.
Albert Einstein

For some people, imagining this may seem a bit overwhelming at first. Or it may seem to be a burden and a responsibility they are not willing or able to take. Balderdash! By the time you finish reading this book, and begin implementing its many common sense suggestions, you will come to realize through your own unique experiences that taking care of the cells of your own body is not only easy and understandable, but totally and completely liberating. The care of your cells is the key to your own personal health and the key to your own personal freedom. You now hold that key. What you do with that key is totally up to you.

Section 1 - Getting Ready

Every manifestation of the life of our tissues, organs and cells, our thoughts, our nerves, our affections, the cruelty, the ugliness, and the beauty of the universe, even its very existence, (all) depend upon the biochemical state of our blood and lymph; and these fluids depend upon the quality of our daily nutrition. Nutrition is synonymous with existence. (Alexis Carrel, *Man the Unknown*, 71)

Russell's Rules for Optimal Digestion

As I like to tell my clients, these rules are not optional, *they are mandatory*. And let's be clear from the outset, these are not "my" rules, they are "the" rules. You must admit, *Russell's Rules* has a nice ring to it. Again, these are not *my rules* and I make no claim to their ownership, invention, or discovery. These are the rules for optimal digestion as they have come down to us through the generations and they represent a very thoughtful and comprehensive system of guidance grounded in traditional wisdom and common sense. These rules are a gift to all of us from our ancestors. The rest of the book goes on to explain *why* these rules are so important but I thought it would be helpful to explain some of them right at the beginning…a kind of preview of coming attractions.

1. If optimal digestion and comfortable elimination is your goal, never restrict your belly with tight-fitting underwear or pants or skirts with tight fitting waistbands. You may think this is silly and obvious, but you would be amazed how many people make how they look more important than how they feel. Wear loose fitting undergarments and loose fitting pants. Your belly will love it and will thank you for paying attention to this important little detail.

2. Think before you eat or drink anything always: "What nourishes me best?"

3. Select the highest quality foods and beverages always. Organic quality is best.

4. Learn how and why to select and prepare your foods and beverages. Find the best whole foods cooking instructors in your area and take some lessons.

5. Give thanks before you eat or drink anything always. Where did this food or beverage come from? Where is it going? Why? Who am I? Why am I here? What nourishes me best? If not me, then who? If not now, then when? Who or what is the ultimate source for all foods and beverages? Who or what is the ultimate source for all human nutrition? One day (several years ago) my son Evan came home from kindergarten and was very excited to share a new *grace before meals* he had just learned in school: *Earth who gives to us this food, sun who makes it ripe and good, dearest earth and dearest sun, we'll not forget what you have done.* Seek grace and grace will find you. Say grace and grace will mind you.

6. Create an atmosphere of peace and quiet, relaxation and calmness around mealtimes. Light a candle. Put on some quiet music. Turn off the TV. Turn off the radio news. Shut off the phone. Shut down your computer. Don't eat when you are angry, upset, stressed out, or tired. First, relax. Go for a walk, clear your head, breathe. Don't let meal time be invaded by other time. Mealtimes are special. Mealtimes are sacred.

7. Always sit down when you eat.

8. Enjoy regular mealtimes. Find balance in your day. Seek harmony in your daily activities. Look to the rhythms in nature and discover how they relate to your life.

9. Eat one mouthful at a time. Put less food on your fork or spoon. Eat less, chew more. Put down your fork, spoon, knife, or chopsticks between mouthfuls. Chew each mouthful until your food becomes liquid. Slow down. Eat less, chew more.

These rules are continued and expanded upon starting on page 157.

Section 1 - Getting Ready

Do You Know Anyone with Digestive System Problems?

There is currently an epidemic of digestive illness in the United States, an epidemic that is directly related to the foods we eat and the way we live. One third to one half of all adults have digestive illness. According to a recent study, 69% of the people studied reported having at least one *gastro-intestinal* problem within the previous three-month period. Except for the common cold, digestive problems are the most common reason people seek medical advice. Digestive problems are the third largest category of illness in the United States today. Some staggering statistics: digestive illness affects at least 62 million Americans per year, resulting in 229 million sick days, at a cost of $41 billion annually and 191,000 deaths. Constipation plagues our nation. The average American spends at least $500 a year on laxatives alone. Zantac*, an ulcer medication, is the best selling drug of all time, with sales in excess of $1 billion annually. (Elizabeth Lipski, *Digestive Wellness* [Los Angeles: Keats Publishing, 2000], 3)

(* In 2006 this distinction probably belongs to Nexium, the little purple pill.)

(* In 2014, Nexium, Prilosec and Prevacid are the big three antacid medications.)

Section 1 - Getting Ready

Do you know anyone with digestive system problems?

Ok, that was a rhetorical question. Of course you know someone with digestive system problems, or you wouldn't be reading this book. I want you to know a few things about me and about the work that I do before I go diving in and giving you specific suggestions to address your digestive system problems. Please be patient. The *need to know* information in the next few pages will be critical in assisting you to gain the levels of confidence and certainty that will ensure your success with this program.

Since 1980, I have helped thousands of people with digestive system problems to learn the dietary and lifestyle habits that result in better digestive system functioning, and in most cases, a rapid return to overall health and well-being. I have a master's degree in Functional Nutrition and Nutrition Counseling. I am pursuing a PhD in the area of gastro-intestinal health. I regularly receive patient referrals from area hospitals and clinics. *I specialize in difficult to solve digestive system problems.* I want to make something very clear to you and I don't want you to take it the wrong way. *You are unique and special but your digestive system problems are not.* They may seem unique and special to you. You may have been told that they are unique and special. You may even have been told that your digestive system problems are *incurable*. You have probably been told that *the cause* of your digestive system problem is *unknown*. I was told these same things forty years ago. I hear it from new clients every single day. It amazes me and concerns me that such misinformation exists. It just isn't true.

What's true is that your digestive system and my digestive system and Aunt Polly's digestive system are basically all the same digestive system: the same anatomical parts and pieces governed and regulated by the same biological laws subject to the same physiological and biochemical dynamics controlled by and determined by the very same dietary and lifestyle habits and influences. The *cause* of your digestive system problems will be found in your dietary and lifestyle choices. Not genetics. Not some hidden, obscure, mysterious, past-life, alien, other-worldly, or otherwise inexplicable *cause*.

How do I know this? Because I have been observing this phenomenon for over 40 years. There is a very important principle in Functional Nutrition called *biochemical individuality,* but this does not mean that the cause of each and every digestive system problem is unique. It means that from a diversity of biochemical configurations and sequencing, there can be, and will be a unity of function. It means that from great complexity, there can be miraculous simplicity. Functional simplicity.

This is very good news. So please stop thinking that your digestive system is so messed up that it is beyond hope and beyond repair. It isn't. What's true is that some digestive systems are worse than yours and some are better than yours. It doesn't matter. What matters is that you start believing that you can take the steps that will heal your digestive system and start to take those steps and continue taking those steps until you are symptom-free, dis-ease free, and totally healed and well again. What you do after that is of course up to you. Imagine that.

What's true is that your digestive system knows exactly how to restore itself to complete and normal functioning (*and then stay that way*), but to do this it requires your cooperation and assistance. And I know that some of you reading this are saying: "What the heck do you think I've been doing, Russell!" I know that many of you have tried "everything." What I can tell you with confidence is this: You probably have uncovered some of the pieces of the puzzle of digestive system health, but not all of the pieces of the puzzle. If you were implementing all of the pieces of the puzzle you would already be healthy and symptom-free, and not looking for solutions in another book. Right?

This book contains all the pieces of the puzzle and it has taken me 40 years to find them. The confidence and certainty you sense from me comes from this belief. This is also one of the reasons I have waited so long to publish this book. I wanted to be absolutely certain I could help everyone (*who wanted to be able to help themselves*) and that includes you! So keep reading and if you haven't already done so, take out a pen or pencil and a hi-liter and start taking notes and writing down your questions, comments, and insights. This is truly the start of something big in your life. I know you have waited a long time for this, and have suffered greatly in the process. I do not take lightly your suffering and your frustration. I take our relationship and its healing potential very seriously, as you will discover.

Section 1 - Getting Ready

Why I Am Writing This Book

I was misdiagnosed with colon cancer in 1973, and even though it turned out to be ulcerative colitis and not cancer, I was very motivated to discover the cause and cure of my own condition. I suffered for seven long years until I finally figured out how to heal myself. You may have suffered that long already, or even longer. I am sorry that you have suffered at all. I am glad you are reading this book. I look forward to hearing from you and having you tell me how effective this program has been in getting you well and keeping you well.

For seven long years I made the same prayer-bargain with God every single night as I tried in vain to get some sleep. I had insomnia, anxiety, and depression for most of the time for most of those seven years alongside my digestive system problems. My prayer-bargain went something like this: "Dear God! If I ever figure out the solution to my digestive system problems, I promise to dedicate the rest of my life to helping other people who find themselves in the same situation that I am in now."

That's why I am writing this book. I made a promise to God and I am keeping that promise. I have been keeping this promise since 1980, since I first started helping other people to heal themselves from various problems, including digestive system problems.

I figured out how to get myself well and keep myself well. And I didn't do it on my own either. Lots of people helped me. And God helped me.

Let me invest a few moments of our time together to talk about God. There are so many possible relationships to the subject of God. I do not want my position about God to be a distraction or impediment in your healing journey and our work together. Whatever your beliefs, I honor them (including no belief in God at all). Whatever your understanding or practice of religion or God or spirituality, or whatever you choose to call it, I honor it. As the poet Rumi once said: "There are hundreds of ways to kneel and kiss the ground." In my teens and early twenties I felt a deep calling to the religious life and seriously considered a vocation as a Roman Catholic monk, or brother. That all changed radically as a result of my own personal healing crisis, many years of gradual recovery, and eventual self-healing.

It would require many pages to describe my own current understanding of religion and spirituality and God. There just isn't time. I don't think you *need to know* these things about me in order for the information in this book to be effective for the purpose of the healing of your own digestive system problems. I have helped people from all walks of life, including every imaginable religious and spiritual persuasion. Your religious beliefs will not prevent you from getting well, unless you are restricted from eating wholesome food, drinking pure water, and breathing fresh, clean air. I simply want you to know that I consider myself to be someone of deep spiritual conviction and faith. I have had many blessings in my life, some that I consider to be miracles.

I believe in God. I believe in God and I am comfortable with knowing that I may never fully understand what that means.

God is an intelligible sphere, whose center is everywhere and circumference, nowhere.
Anonymous

I know that we are not alone. I know that healing is not only possible, but inevitable, if we understand and practice consistently the things that nourish us best. I believe firmly that God wants us to learn how to heal ourselves and then to teach these skills to others. This core belief gives meaning and purpose to my life. I believe that God is a nourishing and benevolent presence: in my life, in your life, and in the world that moves around us and within us. I hope these few thoughts are helpful.

In spite of everything, humanity is still a noble experiment filled with the promise of goodness and grace!
Anonymous

Section 1 - Getting Ready

The information and suggestions in this book are the result of many trial and error experiments over many years, leading edge technology and research, and lots of good-old common sense. I could not begin to name all the people over all the years that have helped me to put the pieces of this puzzle together into the program you are about to discover…so I won't even try. At least not here and now. I will attempt to acknowledge some of these people at the end of the book. I just want to reassure you that this is not something I take lightly, and it most certainly is not some collection of good ideas that might work, or the latest fad, or some new diet, or anything like that. Rest assured that this program works for all the right reasons based upon how your very own digestive system actually functions. This program works *no matter what your digestive system problems are and no matter what your problems have been labeled.* Though I sincerely believe you are an exceptional person, your problems are not the exception to the rules of Functional Nutrition, as you are about to discover. Imagine that.

Section 1 - Getting Ready

The Most Common Digestive System Problems

Here is a short list of the most commonly experienced digestive system problems and/or intestinal disorders: IBS (Irritable Bowel Syndrome), IBD (Inflammatory Bowel Disease), Colitis, Ulcerative Colitis (UC), Crohn's Disease, Colon Cancer, GERD (Gastro-Esophageal-Reflux-Disease). GERD used to be called Acid Reflux, which used to be called Indigestion, which used to be called Heartburn, which used to be called *agita* by my old Italian uncles, and which probably had many similar names in other countries as well. What used to be *heartburn*, and then *acid reflux* has now become *Acid-Reflux-Disease*. I just wanted to mention this because the allopathic treatment of choice for *Acid-Reflux-Disease* is the *little purple pill* called Nexium...with over one billion dollars in annual sales. Imagine that. Ulcers (which can occur anywhere along the entire 30 foot long gastro-intestinal tube which starts at our mouth and ends at the rectum), Hemorrhoids, Hernia, Hiatal Hernia, Gallstones, Constipation, Colonic Inertia, Diarrhea, Gastritis, Gastroparesis, Various GI Infections, Diverticulitis, Diverticulosis, Proctitis, Ulcerative Proctitis, Celiac Disease, Esophagitis, Candida Albicans (which is an opportunistic yeast infection inside the digestive tract), Indigestion, Intestinal Dysbiosis, Intestinal Permeability (aka Leaky Gut Syndrome), SIBO (Small Intestinal Bacteria Overgrowth). I probably missed a few. Let me know if you have a digestive problem whose name is not listed here. Send an email to: russellmariani@healingdigestiveillness.com

Here is another list of some (but not all) of the symptoms and/or conditions directly related to one or more of the "official" intestinal disorders listed above. Notice that some symptoms also appear to be disorders and vice versa. Please also notice that the word disorder simply means *a lack of order* and that the word disease simply means *a lack of ease*. One of the things I love about the Functional Nutrition approach to health, which you will be learning about in the pages of this book, is the way it diffuses and demystifies so many scary looking medical words, terms, and phrases. We need to take the focus off *pathology* and *disease* and *dysfunction*. We need to stop using words like *incurable* and sentences like: *We don't know the cause of this disease.* We need to stop doing this because it simply isn't true anymore. And it never was true. But that is the subject of many other interesting articles, books and programs.

> Western allopathic medicine, seeking only to destroy
> disease causing micro-organisms rather than
> strengthening the person against them,
> is based on a total misconception.
> Sagen Ishizuka

This idea may be hard to swallow. This observation and concept may be difficult to digest. Nevertheless, the simple fact of the matter is this: Whatever label we give to any intestinal disorder and whatever symptoms are related to it, there are many things we can do to restore *order* and *ease* and *normal functioning* to our digestive systems. How? By physically rebuilding our intestines, cell by cell, inch by inch, section by section. This is the process I am calling *intestinal regeneration*. It is based on the concept of restoring normal intestinal function, not by killing pathological organisms alone, but by strengthening the entire body and nourishing our own innate healing capacities.

> We are what we repeatedly do.
> Excellence then, is not an act, but a habit.
> Aristotle

Here is that list of some (but not all) of the symptoms and/or conditions that are directly related to one or more of the "official" intestinal disorders listed above:

Abdominal pain, asthma, chronic joint pain, chronic muscle pain, chronic headaches, migraines, insomnia, dizziness, tinnitus or ringing in the ears, constant coughing, sore throat, hoarseness, swelling/pain in the throat, gagging, frequently clearing the throat, sores on gums, lips, and tongue, mental confusion, fuzzy thinking, poor memory, anger, irritability, binge eating or drinking, poor comprehension, poor concentration, food cravings, difficulty learning, intestinal gas and bloating, indigestion, nausea, vomiting, stomach pain, cramping, heartburn, mood swings, nervousness, diarrhea, poor exercise tolerance, poor immunity, recurrent vaginal infections, bed-wetting, recurrent bladder infections, fevers of unknown origin, shortness of breath, constipation, colonic inertia, aggressive behavior, acute anxiety, easily fatigued, general malaise, chronic fatigue, depression, runny or stuffy nose, postnasal drip, buzzing in the ears, blurred vision, sinus problems, watery and itchy eyes, eye floaters, ear infections, hearing loss, sneezing attacks, hay fever, excessive mucous formation, dark circles under the eyes, swollen, red, or sticky eyelids, irregular heartbeat (palpitations, arrhythmia), rapid heartbeat, chest pain and congestion, bronchitis, shortness of breath, difficulty breathing, hives, skin rashes, psoriasis, eczema, dry skin, oily skin, excessive sweating, excessive body odor, halitosis (bad breath), acne, hair loss, irritation around the eyes, joint weakness, generalized weakness everywhere in the body, muscle aches and pains, arthritis, swelling, stiffness, apathy, pessimism, low self-esteem, hyperactivity, restlessness, overweight, obesity, underweight, anorexia, bulimia, dandruff, fluid retention, genital itch, incontinence, urgent-frequent urination.

Let me know if you are currently suffering from any symptom(s) not listed here: Send an email to: russellmariani@healingdigestiveillness.com

Section 1 - Getting Ready

🌰 What Is "The Cause" of All These Problems?

Since I have made a commitment to you to primarily focus on *need to know* information, I am going to cut to the chase here a bit and distill the millions of pages of books and articles and research reports devoted to answering this question down to a few simple paragraphs. There is no *single cause* for any "degenerative" health problem. There are multiple causes, all working together, preventing your body from functioning normally. These *causes* are various habits and influences in our environment, diet, and lifestyle.

> *We should first exclude the simpler causes*
> *for disease emergence in the body, and then*
> *(and only then!) think of the more complicated causes.*
> Feyerdoon Batmanghelidj, MD

The *root causes* of all digestive system problems are:

Dehydration - (chronic unintentional dehydration)

Nutritional Deficiencies - (especially micro-nutrient deficiencies)

Nutritional Excess - (especially macro-nutrient imbalances)

Dysbiosis - (intestinal dysbiosis)

Stress - (including toxic overload, eating too fast, and many other stress factors)

Let me explain each one briefly.

Root Cause #1
Chronic Unintentional Dehydration

75% of the physical structure of the human body is water. 65% to 85% of the physical structure of every cell in our body is water. Our blood is mostly water; our brain cells, mostly water. Water, as the major component of each and every bodily fluid carries nutrients (including oxygen) to our 100 trillion plus cells, and carries away metabolic waste. Our digestive system needs lots of water to properly process and effectively eliminate our fecal waste matter. *Chronic unintentional dehydration* is one of the root causes of constipation, and almost every other dysfunction in the body as well.

Nothing happens inside our bodies, in terms of basic physiological functions without the presence and assistance of water (including most importantly) digestion!

Everyone knows that you are supposed to drink water. In fact, if you ask Aunt Polly, or even Joe Sixpack, they will tell you that we are supposed to drink at least 8 to 10 eight ounce glasses of water every single day. They will not be able to tell you *why*, but most people have learned this little health-tip along the way. Proper daily hydration is one of the most important *complementary habits* on the road to complete intestinal regeneration.

The truth is, most of us are dehydrated, even if we drink a lot of water! I know this from direct personal experience and I see it confirmed and re-affirmed every single day in the stories told to me by my clients. Even if we drink water, there are many dehydrating influences in our diets and life-styles. Coffee, tea, alcohol, soda, and too much meat and sugar are all dehydrating. Many medications are dehydrating. Exercise is dehydrating. Sitting in an office is dehydrating. Airplane travel is dehydrating. The stress of rush-hour traffic and commuting in general is dehydrating. Even if you sat in bed for the entire day, your body would still sweat one quart of water. Doing nothing is dehydrating!

I have people tell me all the time: "I drink tons of water!" Maybe they do and maybe not.

Drinking water, even drinking a lot of water, does not mean you are properly hydrated. I first learned the difference between *drinking water* and *proper daily hydration* from the world's foremost authority on the subject, Fereydoon Batmanghelidj, MD. He is better known to his many friends and colleagues as Dr. B.

> Water, the solvent of the body, regulates all functions, including the activity of the solutes it dissolves and circulates. Chronic cellular dehydration painfully and prematurely kills. Its initial outward manifestations have until now been labeled as *diseases of unknown origin*. The greatest health discovery of all times is that water is a natural medication for a variety of health conditions. (F.Batmanghelidj, MD, *Your Body's Many Cries for Water* [Falls Church, VA: Global Health Solutions, 1995], 19)

Some of the conditions Dr. B. associates with chronic cellular dehydration include: asthma, allergies, *dyspeptic pain, stomach ulcers, constipation, colitis, hiatal hernia*, rheumatoid arthritis, angina, headaches, migraines, depression, anxiety, insomnia, high blood pressure, hypertension, high cholesterol, obesity, and diabetes among many others.

I first learned about Dr. B and his *watercure recipe* (page 120) back in the winter of 1997. I was suffering from one of the worst periods of depression and anxiety in many years. I was acutely dehydrated and did not realize it. After a long telephone conversation with the good Dr. B, I started to implement the basic ingredients of the watercure recipe into my daily routine. After fourteen days on the watercure my depression lifted and has not returned since. Not once. After 25 years of periodic and medically "unexplainable" depression and anxiety, I was finally free. Nothing else I had tried in all those 25 years worked. And I tried everything. Since the most basic and fundamental *root cause* of my problem was dehydration, the only thing that was going to work in order to reverse, regenerate, and *heal* my condition was to get properly hydrated and then stay properly hydrated.

Imagine that.

It has been 17 years since that pivotal learning experience and I can tell you this. I have not missed one day in all that time of making sure I am properly hydrated. At first I was driven by the fear of the anxiety and depression returning. Now I am motivated by the experience of being well and staying well and understanding the role that proper daily hydration plays in the normal functioning of my body. I follow the watercure recipe precisely, each and every day. It is always my first recommendation to others no matter what the health issue is, but most especially for anyone with digestive system problems.

Note from RM: I update the watercure recipe annually so make sure you have a current copy by checking my website: www.healingdigestiveillness.com

The importance of this *complementary habit* of proper daily hydration cannot be over-stated or over-emphasized. Just like the earth itself, we have our own hydrologic cycle within us, and its fluctuations, modifications, and proper daily maintenance represents one of the most significant opportunities we have to take proactive control of our health and dramatically increase the quality and quantity of our life in the process. I encourage you to jump ahead to page 120 and read the *watercure recipe* and start implementing it right away. There is nothing to lose and everything to gain by doing this.

Here is a summary of some of the most important things I learned about *proper daily hydration* from Dr. B's first book, *Your Body's Many Cries for Water:*

• Dehydration can cause disease. It is often the root cause of many problems.

• Every function of the human body depends on water.

• Morning sickness may be a thirst signal of both fetus and mother.

• The dry mouth is the very last sign of dehydration.

• Products manufactured in the brain cells are transported on waterways to their destination in the nerve endings for use in the transmission of messages.

• Proteins and enzymes in the body function better when the body is hydrated.

• The body needs water! Coffee, tea, fruit juice and other beverages mixed with water don't count. The body needs a certain amount of pure water every single day.

• Proper daily hydration is the key to normal immune system functioning.

Section 1 - Getting Ready

- Your body needs a minimum volume of drinking water each and every day that is roughly half your body weight in ounces. A 200 pound person drinks 100 ounces.

- Dark colored urine is a good sign of serious dehydration. The normal color of urine should be somewhere between very light yellow to almost clear, the color of lite beer.

- Don't overdo it either. Too much water is just as bad as not enough.

- Build up to normal levels gradually. The cells of the body are like sponges. It takes time for them to become properly hydrated again. Allow two to three weeks time.

- Organic sea salt is important to a healthy body. Oxygen, water, sodium, and potassium rank as the primary elements for the survival of the human body. Please avoid commercial table salt which is highly processed and totally denatured.

- Sodium deficiency could be a factor in the development of osteoporosis.

- The water you drink should contain a small amount of organic sea salt to aid in the absorption and assimilation of the water and minerals into your cells. About one quarter of a teaspoon per quart is all that is needed. If this tastes too strong at first, start with a smaller amount (even one grain of salt) and build up gradually.

- If you drink 100 ounces of water per day, you will eliminate 100 ounces of urine. This is normal. Whatever volume of water you drink you can expect to produce an equal volume of urine. The frequency of urination may increase, but the urgency should feel normal. Your bladder capacity will expand (and return to normal size and shape) as it becomes properly hydrated again.

- Urinary incontinence is often caused by a condition of chronic unintentional dehydration.

The habit of proper daily hydration is a huge piece of the puzzle in our *Intestinal Regeneration Program*. You will want to re-read the above quotations several times and really think about them. Most importantly, you will want to integrate the habit of proper daily hydration via the *watercure recipe* as soon as possible. There are other habits, as you will discover, that are equally important, but there is no habit more important than proper daily hydration. Purchase and read Dr. B's books about hydration and health. You will find more information about this and other topics in the *Resources* section at the end of the book.

Root Cause #2
Nutritional Deficiencies
(especially micro-nutrient deficiencies)

There are two major categories of nutrients; macronutrients and micronutrients. Macronutrients are proteins, carbohydrates, fats, and fiber. Micronutrients include things like vitamins, minerals, trace-minerals, enzymes, amino acids, essential fatty acids, phyto-nutrients, anti-oxidants, and pigments like chlorophyl. Most people get enough macronutrients in their diet. They may eat too much protein, too many carbohydrates and too much fat, but deficiencies in macronutrients is not usually the problem in the United States and other developed countries. Macronutrient deficiency is a very serious problem in Third World countries. Any time you hear or see stories about starvation, you are seeing the long term results of macronutrient deficiencies. Where there is macronutrient deficiency, there is always micronutrient deficiency. The problem in the United States and other modern and industrialized nations is primarily micronutrient deficiencies (along with the other major causes of degenerative disease).

Why aren't we getting the micronutrients we need?

We eat too many processed foods.

We eat too much snack food, junk food, chips, candy, and chocolate bars. We drink too much soda, coffee, tea, beer, wine, and other alcoholic beverages. We don't drink enough water. We eat too many foods made from the flour milled from whole grains and not the whole grains themselves. Bread, muffins, pastries, donuts, chips, pretzels, cookies, cakes, pies, cereals, pasta are all processed foods made from refined and processed grains. We eat too many processed luncheon meats. We eat too many processed breakfast cereals. We eat too many previously prepared foods. We eat too many frozen and bottled and canned foods and not enough fresh foods. We do not eat enough whole foods. For a complete list of whole foods and processed foods read the article called: *The Modern Cornucopia*. (page 182)

Let me attempt to permanently clarify the critical distinction between whole grain foods and processed foods that are made from the milling of whole grains. (*The Truth About Whole Grains* is found on page 187.) The milling process turns whole grains into flour. Whole grains are seeds. You wash them, put them in a pot with water, bring them to a boil then simmer them for about an hour. This basic gruel or porridge has served as a staple food for thousands of years in many cultures around the world. As seeds, you can put whole grains in soil and in a few days they will sprout. This is the only relevant test of whether you have a whole grain in front of you or some processed food made from the milling of whole grains. You can't put a rolled oat or corn flake or rice puff in the soil and have it sprout. Why? Because these are not whole grains! They are highly processed foods made from the flour of whole grains (or in the case of rolled oats, simply flattened in a stainless steel roller).

The best way to get the full nutritional benefits from whole grains is to eat them in a cooked, whole form. This is a distinction of critical importance for the success of your *Intestinal Regeneration Program*. (Specific guidelines for the preparation of cooked whole cereal grains will be found on pages 149 and 234) Almost every form of processed whole grain product is, at best, nutritionally weak and at worst, nutritionally worthless. Processed grain products are not neutral. Processed grain products in the diet are one of the primary causes of all digestive system problems!

Why aren't we getting the micronutrients we need? We *over*cook our foods, destroying many heat-sensitive micronutrients and enzymes. We microwave foods, permanently altering molecular structures and also destroying heat-sensitive nutrients. We harvest fruits and vegetables prematurely and ripen them artificially in refrigerated trucks. We add things to our foods like preservatives, coloring agents, artificial sugars, artificial flavor enhancers, antibiotics, growth hormones and genetically modified organisms (GMOs). The presence of these non-essential and non-nutrient substances interferes with the normal intake of micronutrients from our bloodstream and into our cells.

Many of the substances I just listed are toxic to the body and cause additional stresses and strains. Please read the article called: *Toxicology and Human Health* (page 189) to better assess the damage to our bodies caused by these various non-nutrient substances. As far as our body is concerned, if the substance or fluid in question is not helpful to normal cellular functioning, then it's harmful. If it is not nutritious to the body, it's toxic to the body. Nothing is neutral. It's just this simple.

Another *cause* of nutritional deficiencies has to do with the lack of minerals and trace minerals in the soils themselves. The Green Revolution in modern agriculture started right after World War II with the implementation of NPK fertilizers. NPK stands for Nitrogen (N), Potassium (P), and Phosphorus (K). It was initially accepted that applying only these three minerals to the soil would be sufficient for optimal growing conditions for all of our food crops. But the soil scientists were sadly mistaken. As it turns out, dozens of minerals are needed to be present in the soil, along with dozens of various soil micro-organisms and soil bacteria and enzymes and earthworms and other things in order for food plants to absorb and then manufacture the nutrients that we depend upon for health.

> A few of the trace minerals necessary for healthy plant growth are: magnesium, zinc, iron, copper, calcium, boron, manganese, molybdenum, cobalt, and chromium. But the absence of just one element (mineral) from the soil can cause great health problems. For instance, if inorganic cobalt is missing from the soil, the plant cannot absorb it and convert it into organic cobalt. Without organic cobalt, the human body cannot manufacture vitamin B12. When we don't get enough vitamin B12, we can't assimilate iron properly or make strong red blood cells. If we can't make strong red blood cells, we become anemic. Anemic people become weak, depressed, and vulnerable to disease. (Dr. Bernard Jensen, *Empty Harvest* [New York City: Avery Publishing Group, 1990], 8)

The primary reason to make the shift away from conventionally grown food crops (including conventionally raised and processed animal food products) towards organically grown food crops is that organic farmers invest heavily in building mineral-rich and micro-organism-rich soil, and conventional farmers do not. *If the minerals are not in the soil, they simply cannot show up in our food plants.* It's just this simple. Organic farmers avoid the use of toxic fertilizers, pesticides, herbicides, fungicides, antibiotics, preservatives, growth hormones and GMOs, but conventional farmers, growers, and processors do not avoid these harmful influences and production methods. They are starting to. *Clean food* is a buzz phrase today and the fastest growing trend in the *billions of dollars* food business.

Certified Organic is your only insurance of truly clean food and beverage products. (*How To Find Certified Organic Foods* is found on page 194.)

Finally, we suffer from nutritional deficiencies when the villi and micro-villi in our small intestines (our literal internal root system) are not functioning properly. Most commonly, our villi and micro-villi are not functioning properly because the balance between beneficial bacteria and pathological bacteria is off. This is a condition called *intestinal dysbiosis*. (Read about this in Root Cause #4 below.)

Root Cause #3
Nutritional Excess
(especially macro-nutrient imbalances)

Too many people eat too much food: too much protein, too much refined carbohydrates, too much fat.

Imagine that.

We consume too much processed food; too much party food, snack food, junk food. We eat too fast. We eat too often. We eat too much. When the digestive system is stressed from overwork, instead of converting our food nutrients to energy (its primary function), it converts our food nutrients to fat. We must chew more and eat less.

We must find the correct balance between and among protein, carbohydrate and fatty foods. We must eat more whole foods and eat less processed foods. We must eat less and chew more. More about this important *root cause* will be discussed throughout the rest of the book.

Section 1 - Getting Ready

🌰 Root Cause #4
Intestinal Dysbiosis

Ninety-nine percent of all the world's bacteria is helpful and beneficial to life in general and human beings in particular. Over 400 individual strains of beneficial bacteria have so far been identified as useful inhabitants of the human digestive system. Imagine that.

The two most popular and beneficial intestinal bacteria are called bifidus and acidophilus. Beneficial intestinal bacteria are commonly known by the name *probiotics*. Biotics comes from biology, which is the study of life or the study of living organisms. The prefix *pro* means "for" or "in support of." Thus, the word probiotics means *for life* or *in support of life*. Acidophilus is the dominant probiotic in the small intestine. Bifidus is the dominant probiotic in the large intestine. There are other probiotic materials, but none are more important than these two.

In 1908, Dr. Eli Metchnicoff won the Nobel Prize for medicine for his work on the role of probiotics and their ability to boost the human immune system He was a colleague of Louis Pasteur and succeeded him as the director of the Pasteur Institute in Paris. He coined the term *dysbiosis* as a way of describing a condition that was opposite one of intestinal *symbiosis*, which means living together in a state of mutual balance and harmony. The prefix, dys means *not*, so dysbiosis describes a condition of intestinal imbalance, conflict and turbulence...even outright war. And it certainly feels like a war going on down there, doesn't it?

Dysbiosis or Intestinal Dysbiosis refers to the imbalance of intestinal bacteria, sometimes referred to generally as the intestinal microflora. When the intestinal bacteria are out of balance, the entire list of digestive system problems, symptoms, conditions, disorders, and labeled diseases become increasingly more likely to the point of inevitability. One of the most common problems associated with intestinal dysbiosis is the overgrowth of a very nasty opportunistic bacteria/yeast called candida albicans. This is usually referred to as a "yeast infection." It is also known as candidiasis.

Other problems associated with intestinal dysbiosis are these: intestinal permeability or leaky gut syndrome, mal-absorption syndrome, chronic fatigue, dizziness, the inability to concentrate, gastritis, abdominal cramping, flatulence, constipation, diarrhea, and skin problems including acne. This is a very short list. Go back a few pages and realize that every single digestive symptom/condition listed there is in some way directly related to the problem of intestinal dysbiosis.

The bottom line is this *when pathological bacteria exist in the gut they produce toxins that cause symptoms of ill health and dis-ease.*

When the intestinal bacteria are out of balance you will have symptoms and you will be sick, and nothing you try will correct this problem completely until you actually correct the *root cause* of the problem. The root cause of intestinal dysbiosis is the imbalance between pathological bacteria and beneficial bacteria. Fortunately the solution is simple. Stop doing the things that kill the beneficial bacteria and invite the increased growth of the pathological bacteria. Start doing the things that nourish and grow the beneficial bacteria and kill the pathological bacteria. Start using effective probiotic supplements every single day to increase the populations of the beneficial bacteria.

Read about **Why Probiotic Supplements Are So Important** on page 217.

Note from RM: At a Healthcare Symposium I attended in 2013 I first heard the term, **The Human Microbiome** in reference to the intestinal flora. Keep in mind that bacteria are not the only types of pathological micro-organisms found in our gut. Viruses, yeast, mold, fungi, parasites, worms and who knows what else may also take up residence in our gut and cause health problems. Maintaining a healthy balance of probiotic materials in the human gut is one of the most important things we can do for our health.

Root Cause #5
Stress

You can easily make the argument that everything in our lives is stressful. It's true. So stress is not the problem. The problem is *the balance* between positive stress factors and negative stress factors. The problem is in not knowing the difference between positive stress factors and negative stress factors. The problem is thinking and believing that negative stress factors are neutral (or relatively neutral as in the phrase "not that bad") and that positive stress factors aren't that important. Nothing could be further from the truth.

First of all, nothing we do and no influence in our diet or lifestyle is neutral.

This may be the single most important sentence in the entire book, so I think I will repeat it: *Nothing we do and no influence in our diet or lifestyle is neutral.*

Every habit, every influence is positive or negative, helpful or harmful. The problem is having too many negative stress factors in our diet and lifestyle and not enough positive stress factors. In all future references in this book, I will be referring to positive stress factors as **complementary** habits and influences and to negative stress factors as **insulting** habits and influences.

For a complete list of these habits and influences as they relate to problems of the digestive system please read: ***The Habits of Functional Nutrition*** on page 157.

Our bodies cannot function normally if we are suffering from micro-nutrient deficiencies. Our bodies cannot function normally if we overwork our digestive system by eating too much and eating too fast. Our bodies cannot function normally if we are dehydrated. Our bodies cannot function normally if we are suffering from intestinal dysbiosis. Our bodies cannot function normally if toxic chemicals and other toxic substances in the environment are finding their way into our cells through our food, water, and air supplies.

The subject of *toxic overload* is critical to a fuller understanding of the relationships between human health and the various environments in which we live and from which we derive all of our sources of sustenance. The presence of microscopic bits of toxic and non-nutritious materials in the body creates the opportunity for cellular malfunction and cellular degeneration. When this process takes root, the door swings open to the possibilities of every degenerative disease symptom and condition known.

> So far 51 chemicals, many of them widely used, have been shown to act at extremely low levels as hormone disrupters in wildlife, laboratory animals, and in humans. Examples include dioxins, (the result of incinerating chlorine-containing products) PCB's, chemicals in many plastics, pesticides, mercury, and lead. Typically, 10-40 years may elapse between the initial exposure to a toxic chemical and the appearance of any detectable symptoms. Partly because of this time-lag, many healthy teenagers and young adults have trouble believing that their smoking, drinking, eating junk foods, and other lifestyle habits today, could lead to some form of degeneration later on. (G. Tyler Miller, ed., *Living in the Environment* [Pacific Grove: CA Brooks/Cole Publishers, 2000], 442)

---

*For the first time in the history of the world,
every human being is now subjected to dangerous chemicals
from the moment of conception until death.*
Rachel Carson

🌰 Is There a "Cure" For All These Problems?

The word "cure" has a lot of baggage attached to it. The modern allopathic medical-pharmaceutical-industrial-research *complex* has invested billions and billions of dollars to find *the cure* for all the digestive disorders already mentioned and every other known sickness and disease as well. The result of all those billions of dollars invested? Degenerative Disease is now the number one cause of death in America today and has been for the last thirty or forty years.

Imagine that.

The physician is only the servant of nature, not her master. Therefore, it behooves medicine, to follow the will of nature.
Paracelsus

There is no question that the primary tools of allopathic medicine are pharmaceutical drugs and surgery. If they are not successful in killing disease causing organisms with radiation, chemotherapy, antibiotics, and other biochemical agents, they go to the knife. *When in doubt, cut it out!* Allopathic medicine gives lip service to nutritional and life-style changes, but relies on a vast pharmaceutical armada to stimulate or depress, trick and cajole the cells of the body to do its bidding. At what price? Adverse reactions to normal dosages of common pharmaceuticals are responsible for upwards of 100,000 deaths per year in the United States alone. *The short-term goal of alleviating symptoms has been sacrificed on the altar of quick-fix solutions and corporate greed.* Health should not be defined as the absence of disease symptoms. Health is the presence of vitality. Health cannot be created by alleviating the symptoms of disease but only by nourishing the roots of life within us.

The tissue of life to be, we weave with colors all our own, and in the field of destiny, we reap what we have sown.
John Greenleaf Whittier

Many people are abandoning the religion of false hopes embodied by the phrase *medical cure*. It's about time. I try to remember what my friend and colleague Jeanne Silk once taught me many years ago: "There are only two things in life that have ever been cured; ham and leather."

As a result, I prefer the word "heal" and I like to talk about the process of personal healing. Personal healing is a direct consequence of taking more personal responsibility for our own choices and decisions *and our own results*. So I won't be using the word cure *at all* because I do not want to be associated with pharmaceutical or medical "cures." I make this choice for all kinds of interesting reasons, some of which I can explain easily, others not so easily.

A lot of people do not understand that allopathic medicine is focused on finding medical cures, to the exclusion of almost everything else. (Why aren't we being taught about the benefits of probiotics and their immune boosting capabilities?) Right now, medical cures are defined as pharmaceutical or surgical or biotech interventions. If it cannot be patented, it will not be pursued and we will not hear about it (*it* being anything outside of conventional allopathic medicine). If we do hear about *it*, we will be told that *it* is non-scientific, or anecdotal, or unproven. We will be told that *it* is dangerous and risky.

Many people fail to understand this point. Many people fail to understand that medicine is big business. Because of the triumph of modern medicine over certain contagious diseases like smallpox, tuberculosis, and polio by the middle of the twentieth century, it was assumed that modern medicine would be able to triumph over every other form of disease as well. Maybe it will, but not without some serious revisioning and refocusing and reprioritizing.

More and more physicians will give lip service to the benefits of dietary and lifestyle changes, but they will be very limited as to the best way to help you, the patient, make an effective transition. You probably already know just how true this is, from your own direct personal experience.

What I am presenting in this book is common sense information that just happens to be backed up by the most current and accurate understanding of the anatomy and physiology of the human body and the human digestive system. *Why this information has not filtered down into current allopathic medical practice is not the subject of this book or the purpose of my life.* I am not primarily interested in changing the medical establishment or standard allopathic medical practices although clearly massive changes need to take place. I am primarily interested in helping you to improve the quality of your life, by changing and improving the habits in your diet and your lifestyle. I am primarily interested in helping you to heal yourself. I prefer to use the term *heal*. I will not be using the term *cure* at all in any reference to the purposes of Functional Nutrition in general and to my *Intestinal Regeneration Program* in particular.

Trust me when I tell you that this is not just a matter of mere semantics. Good people have been shut down, shut up, and imprisoned because they did not understand or respect the legal ramifications and political and economic volatility of the critical differences between *medical cures* and *personal, proactive, nutritional healing.*

I healed myself from a variety of digestive system disorders. I healed myself from a 25 year history of panic disorders, anxiety attacks, and periodic bouts of severe, acute clinical depression. I healed myself from these disorders without the use of any pharmaceutical medications or surgical procedures. I healed myself with the proper use of simple whole foods, cellular detoxification and cleansing strategies, effective nutritional supplements, and proper daily hydration. I am writing this book to teach you how to do the same thing, *if you want to!* I am writing this book to teach you how to become more proactive in your own self-care. I believe that you will be able to *heal yourself* from whatever digestive system problem you may be currently suffering. Imagine that.

Let's keep these important differences and distinctions in mind as we move further down the path of personal nutritional healing in general and intestinal regeneration in particular.

What Is Functional Nutrition?

Functional Nutrition is the term I use to describe a set of very specific biological principles at work inside our bodies and in evidence in the natural world around us. It is also a very specific set of complementary dietary and lifestyle habits that, when practiced consistently, have the ability to restore normal functioning to the human body. Normal internal functioning is the first and most basic definition of health according to the rules of Functional Nutrition.

Here is a simple explanation I share with all my clients in the first few days of their *Intestinal Regeneration Program*.

The human body is a marvelously designed living organism with the ability to grow, regulate, repair, and defend itself when given organic quality, full spectrum, whole food nutrition.

This means that: *A well-nourished body doesn't make mistakes.* A well-nourished body is capable of protecting itself from sickness and disease and fully capable of producing all the symptoms of health: energy, flexibility, creativity, optimism, compassion, laughter, cooperation, vision, wisdom, and more. Creating a well-nourished body requires our personal commitment to self-healing, our conscious attention to the details in our diet and lifestyle, and our proactive participation in the habits that nourish us best. I call this approach to health, Functional Nutrition.

Here's how it works:

The quality of our physical health is determined by the quality of the life of our cells.

Section 1 - Getting Ready

Each and every human body is composed of trillions and trillions of cells. Each cell is like a little factory (page 195). Each cell requires very specific nutrients or raw materials. Each cell produces products essential to our overall metabolism and health. Each cell produces toxic waste products that must be neutralized and eliminated on a continual basis. Our cells compose the tissues, which compose the organs, which compose the systems that make up the whole human body. *Our cells constitute the biological foundation of our lives.* There is nothing more important in the process of regaining, maintaining, or improving the quality of our physical health than taking proper care of our cells. Health is the result of the proper care of our cells.

> Each cell continually synthesizes and dissolves structures and eliminates waste products. Tissues and organs replace their cells in continual cycles. There is growth, development and evolution. The function of each cellular component is to participate in the production or transformation of other components within the cell and within the entire cellular network. In this way, the network continually makes itself. It is produced by its components and in turn produces those components.
> (Fritjof Capra, *The Web of Life* [New York City: Doubleday, 1996], 159)

> Every manifestation of the life of our tissues, organs and cells, our thoughts, our nerves, our affections, the cruelty, the ugliness, and the beauty of the universe, even its very existence depend upon the biochemical state of our blood and lymph; and these fluids depend upon the quality of our daily nutrition. Nutrition is synonymous with existence. (Alexis Carrel, *Man The Unknown*, 71)

When the cells of our body are functioning properly, our biological foundation is strong and we thrive. When the cells of our body are not functioning properly, our biological foundation is weak and we suffer.

Much of this suffering is preventable and correctable through the daily practice of better and *more complementary* nutrition habits.

The proverbial "gaps" in everyone's biological foundation fall into three categories:

1. *Nutrition Gaps*
2. *Information Gaps*
3. *Integrity Gaps*

Nutrition Gaps are caused by eating too many junk foods and processed foods and not enough organic quality whole foods. Nutrition Gaps are caused by the inefficient processing and digesting of the foods we do consume. Nutrition Gaps are caused from the ineffective use of nutritional supplements, or the non-use of effective supplements. Nutrition Gaps are caused by the practice of too many insulting habits and not enough complementary habits in our diet and lifestyle. Nutrition Gaps show up in our biological foundations after years of nutritional deficiencies, toxic overload, dehydration and stress.

Information Gaps are caused by the constant flow of misinformation from print, radio, television, internet and other sources. Billions of advertising dollars try to persuade us to eat this food, or drink that beverage, or use this medicine. These billions of advertising dollars are *corporate* advertising dollars. These corporations have a binding mandate to generate profit, not human health. Put 100 health and nutrition "experts" in a room and you will get 100 different opinions about what constitutes the ideal human diet. What is the result of all this misinformation? Uncertainty. The constant flow of misinformation has caused a massive river of doubt. This uncertainty and doubt erodes our confidence and is at the *root cause* of so much suffering in our world today. Look at how much stress is caused by the uncertainty about what to eat and what not to eat and why. Do you think our ancestors a few generations ago were so constantly confused and set upon by so many experts about the connections between their food and their health? Not a chance. It is a travesty of unprecedented scope and scale that educated adult human beings are confused about what to eat and why. If this situation weren't so tragic, it would be funny.

Throughout history, most people have not been in conflict on a daily basis about what to eat and why. They may have suffered from a lack of food, but not from a lack of knowledge about what foods to eat and what foods to avoid. Food was food! By and large people ate what was available to them according to the harvest season, their specific geographic location, and their particular ethnic traditions and cuisine. That's the way it has been for at least the past ten thousand years, since the dawn of civilization. What we call civilization begins with the seasonal planting, growing, and harvest of whole grains, root vegetables, and other staple foods. Culture begins with agri-culture.

Today, all of that has changed. Our modern scientific and multi-cultural marketplace of ideas, goods, and services has simply given us too many choices. Nobody seems capable of creating agreement on the topic of what to eat and why. This uncertainty runs contrary to one of our deepest and most basic of all human instincts and emotions: the desire to nurture ourselves and others through food. This uncertainty creates negative stress at a very deep level of our being. I believe it is a stress that rarely gets identified. As a result, it eats away at us, as all negative stress does and we begin to manifest the ill-effects of a kind of strange internal erosion, leading to gaps in our physical, emotional, psychological and spiritual foundations.

Integrity Gaps are caused when we actually know what to do to be healthier, but we don't do it! We know we should exercise more regularly. We know we should eat more slowly, chew better, not eat late at night. We know we should not drink so much coffee and alcohol. Since we are weakened by the ill-effects of Nutrition Gaps on the one hand and Information Gaps on the other, is it any wonder? It is difficult to maintain discipline and integrity in the area of diet and nutrition when you are feeling overfed, undernourished, misinformed, uncertain, stressed-out, and more than a little bit frustrated about the whole subject of nutrition and health.

The purpose of our work together in the days and weeks ahead is to learn what habits and influences in our diet and lifestyle have caused the gaps in our own biological foundation to occur, and then to take the corrective actions to restore them. By doing this we will make our biological foundations healthy and strong and whole again. This is the purpose of the Functional Nutrition approach to health. This is the program of *intestinal regeneration* described in this book. To facilitate this ongoing process of learning and doing we will focus our attention in two key areas:

1. Biological principles which regulate the functions of our physiology, and

2. The habits in our diet and lifestyle which either complement or insult these principles and basic functions.

Section 1 - Getting Ready

Biological Principle Number One: Homeostasis

Homeostasis is the term which describes the dynamic mechanisms within the human body which maintain constant conditions and regulate all internal functions; the beating of our heart, the production of saliva, enzymes and hormones, the healing of cuts and bruises, the oxygenation of cells, the expiration of carbon dioxide from our lungs, the production of insulin and cholesterol, the pH of our blood, the peristaltic motions of our small and large intestines, the constancy of our internal body temperature, etc.

Homeostasis is the miracle of balance and harmony that exists inside every cell, tissue, organ and system of the human body. Homeostasis is the natural intelligence within our own body that knows exactly what to do, to get us well and keep us well. Homeostasis is most evident, most inspiring and perhaps, most astonishing when we observe the inner workings of our little cellular factories: our cells.

> Our bodies; and every organ, tissue, and system within our bodies, *build themselves* from single cells, and renew themselves through the constant interchange of food, water and air. We can say that our bodies are like temples, or like houses, in that houses are made from bricks, and bodies are made from cells, but the comparison would fall far short of the miraculous truth. For our body is born from one cell, as if the house could be built from one brick...a magic brick that would set about manufacturing other bricks. These new bricks, without waiting for the architect's drawings or the arrival of the brick-layers, would somehow assemble themselves and begin to form walls and floors and ceilings. These magical bricks would

also metamorphose into window panes, roofing-slates, coal for heating, and water for the kitchen and bathroom. Our bodies develop by means such as those attributed to fairies in the tales told to children in bygone times. This magnificent construction of our bodies emanates from the unknowable wisdom inside each individual cell, which, to all appearances, possesses a knowledge of the future edifice and synthesizes from substances present in our blood and lymph, not only the building materials, but the workers themselves! (Alexis Carrel, *Man the Unknown*, 92)

We've learned a lot about cells since Alexis Carrel was looking down his microscope in 1935. "Unknowable wisdom inside each individual cell" is not a phrase we are accustomed to hearing from our current science and medical writers. The attitude is always; "We know so much, and what we don't know, we will soon." As we collectively unravel the human genome and attempt other monumental projects, it might be a good idea to maintain some humility. We may never know everything there is to know about the inner workings of cells. Then again, we may not have to. I see people every day heal themselves from all kinds of "incurable" digestive disorders, without the slightest need to fully understand what is actually going on. Sometimes an accurate general description is enough, combined with a healthy dose of humility and some traditional awe. If anything in our lives deserves the adjective *awesome*, it would have to be in reference to our cells.

Our job is to cooperate with the miraculous cells inside our own body and to do the things that nourish us best. The principle of homeostasis teaches us that nothing is neutral. Everything we do, eat, drink, think, and say is either complementary to our homeostasis and health, or it is insulting, and actively destructive to our health.

I repeat: nothing is neutral. Everything is either complementary or insulting to the proper care, design and function of the human body.

Knowing the difference between which influences in our lives are complementary and which influences are insulting is one of the most important things we will ever learn. Practicing the complementary habits and avoiding or minimizing the insulting habits is the surest path to the experience of better health in general and to the experience of *intestinal regeneration* in particular. In Section Two, I will describe in some detail the list I have compiled so far of the most important complementary and insulting habits. You will find this information in the section called: *The Habits of Functional Nutrition*. (page 157)

Complementary Habit Number One: Be Proactive!

Being proactive means taking more complete personal responsibility for our own actions and our own results. It is the most important choice we can make, and we need to make it and remake it, every day of our lives. I believe it is easier to make this choice and remake this choice with a deeper and clearer understanding and appreciation of how the human body works. In particular how cells work, as we have just seen. Aren't the cells of the human body amazing? Of course they are! When the fog of confusion and uncertainty hanging over our own personal river of doubt clears, we find ourselves not only knowing what to do to nourish ourselves best, but eager and happy to do it. We know what the alternatives are! Right?

> *I don't think what people are looking for is the meaning of life. I think what people are looking for is the experience of being more fully alive!*
> Joseph Campbell

Being proactive is a cornerstone of the Functional Nutrition paradigm. Functional Nutrition is a reference to the foods, supplements, and habits that, working together, restore normal physiological functions in our body. This results in the experience of vitality, energy and health. Functional Nutrition reminds us that no one will ever know your own body better than you. Being proactive means that we live our lives in a constant spirit of experimentation and choice; learning by doing. What we need to learn are the complementary habits that nourish us best. What we need to do is to practice them consistently and gradually, master them. Health is the result of this exciting and never-ending process. Your successful *Intestinal Regeneration Program* depends upon your understanding of and your commitment to this transformational educational process.

Section 1 - Getting Ready

Functional Nutrition and the Period of Adjustment

Rome was not built in a day. Your digestive system did not get into its current condition in the past 24 hours. It has taken months and in some cases years for all your insulting habits to catch up with you and manifest into your current condition and symptoms. You will not be able to heal yourself from these symptoms overnight. However, it will not take you years either, and in most cases, not even months. Most of my clients report serious and dramatic improvement within the first few days of following my suggestions as outlined in this *Intestinal Regeneration Program*. However, you must understand something very important before you get started. *Just because your symptoms may lessen in intensity or even disappear altogether, doesn't mean you have completely healed yourself.* Healing takes time. Cellular regeneration takes time. Give yourself at least three to six months on this program and you will be well on your way to an entirely regenerated digestive system that will loyally serve you disease-free for the rest of your life, as long as you continue to cooperate and provide your digestive system the things that it needs to function normally...as long as you serve your digestive system the things that nourish it best!

Exercising your proactive nutrition muscles will make you healthy and strong. There is no question about this. The question you need to ask yourself is this: What condition are my proactive nutrition muscles in right now? Here's what I mean. When you upgrade your nutritional status by implementing this *Intestinal Regeneration Program*, you simultaneously initiate a *biological period of adjustment* inside every cellular factory in the body. This causes your whole body to change, as in improve and get better. The cells of your body will start functioning

Section 1 - Getting Ready

better. This means that metabolic and other toxins are purged, cellular damage is repaired, and normal productivity is restored. Better health results when normal cellular functioning returns. This of course is the whole point.

If your proactive nutrition muscles are already very healthy and strong, you probably will not be reading this book! If your proactive nutrition muscles are new, or relatively unexercised, you could experience some minor physical discomfort until the transitional cleansing and repair work is complete. This could last for as little as a few hours, to a few days, or even a few weeks. This is what I call *the biological period of adjustment*.

The normal functions of detoxification, cleansing and repair going on inside the cells of our body become more effective and sometimes more noticeable when we improve our own nutritional status. This phenomenon is completely normal and very desirable. Practicing more complementary habits, especially the habit of proper daily hydration will decrease the time and minimize any discomfort during the period of adjustment.

This biological period of adjustment I am describing is sometimes referred to generally as a process of detoxification and cleansing. I prefer to use the term *period of adjustment* because although detoxification and cleansing are going on inside our cells, they are not the only things going on inside our cells. Restoration, regeneration, repair and healing are going on as well.

Also, some people panic when they hear the term *detoxification*. Some writers and practitioners use the term *healing crisis* to describe this period of adjustment. I don't like that term either. The crisis is over, the minute you decide to do the things that nourish you best. This period of adjustment represents the most important *opportunity* your body has had in years, perhaps ever; why refer to it as a crisis?

Remember: A well-nourished body doesn't make mistakes. Be patient. Take one step at a time. Your body is a garden. Think of all the work that goes on underground before we see those very first green shoots of spring. The period of adjustment is like spring cleaning going on inside your body. When complete you will look and feel like a new person, but during the process you may look and feel like somebody else entirely! Whatever you experience, it will all be the result of better nutritional choices and better overall internal functioning. Remember: A well-nourished body doesn't make mistakes.

Imagine that.

Section 1 - Getting Ready

Giving Thanks for Our Food

Our body is a garden. This is not a metaphor. It's a fact. The food we eat, the water and beverages we drink, and the air we breathe, literally become the soil of our blood and lymph from which every cell in our body receives its daily sustenance. We are the cultivators of our own inner soil. We provide the nutrients. We reject the poisons. We make the choices as to what comes in and what goes out and why. Each cell in our body is a seed. It is entirely up to us how these seeds turn out. Will they blossom into the ripeness of their full potential? Or will they never know the experience of their own magnificence? As we sow, so shall we reap. Our daily habits determine our health. *Food is the soil from which the tree of our own life is grown.* I am grateful for the garden that is my own body, and for the food which nourishes all the blossomings in my life.

Russell Mariani
November 22, 2001

🌰 A Quick Tour through the Digestive System

Here is some basic *need to know* information about the various parts that make up our digestive system and how they function. The purpose of this tour is to motivate and inspire you to take the suggestions and recommendations in Section Two more seriously. I believe that when you understand just how important (if not miraculous) your digestive system really is, you will take better care of it.

If ignorance is the cause of all human suffering then education is the very best remedy.
Michio Kushi

- The process of digestion begins with the mere sight of food, sometimes with the mere thought of food; sometimes with the smell, fragrance, and aroma of food. Sometimes the process begins out of habit. If we eat lunch at the same time every day, our stomach is conditioed to receive food at a certain time, and if the food doesn't show up on time, we hear about it (rumble, rumble). The increased amount of fluid that you feel in your mouth is the result of an increased production of saliva, which contains digestive enzymes. The increased production of saliva is a physiological response to food, real or imagined. This sets the entire digestive process in motion.

- The mouth: All carbohydrates are digested in the mouth. This is really important. Think about the last time you ate some corn on the cob. Did you see evidence of any incomplete chewing the following day, in the toilet bowl? If you do not chew certain whole

Section 1 - Getting Ready

The Human Digestive System

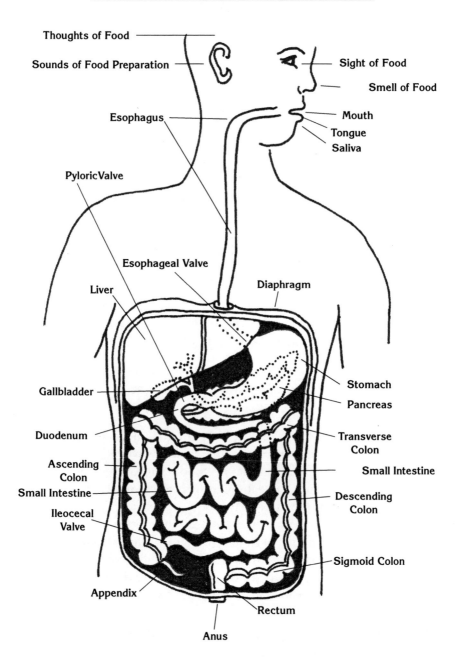

Eat Less - Chew More

foods like whole grains, seeds and certain nuts, they will not get broken down anywhere else. If they are not broken down and turned into liquid (called chyme) the nutrients they contain will not be assimilated and utilized. Nothing is neutral. Improperly digested food causes all kinds of digestive system problems. To be well, we must chew well. Chewing is not optional, it's mandatory.

- The mouth: Saliva contains the digestive enzyme, salivary amylase. This enzyme is designed to break down and liquefy complex carbohydrates, like rice, oats, barley and corn. Our saliva is slightly alkaline. The more we chew the more alkaline our saliva becomes. The better we chew the less hydrochloric acid the stomach has to produce. The more we chew, the easier it is for the next stage of digestion. In fact, the more we chew the easier it is for all the stages of digestion. *To be well we must chew well.* The easiest remedy for all symptoms of acid-reflux is to slow down and chew better.

- The esophagus: The esophagus is a narrow, fleshy tube that connects the back of the mouth or top of our throat to our stomach. Rhythmic muscular waves or contractions usher the (well-chewed) food down the esophagus into our stomach. At the bottom of our esophagus is a fleshy valve called the esophageal valve. This valve is the main victim when a combination of factors produces excess stomach acid. When this valve is not able to contain the stomach contents below, it feels like a burning sensation. Since its physical location is directly behind the heart, we call this sensation heartburn. The technical term is acid-reflux. And now we have acid-reflux-disease.

- Acid-reflux disease occurs after weeks or months of simple but irritating episodes of acid-reflux or heartburn succeed in altering the delicate lining of the esophagus above the esophageal valve. This alteration can feel like a sore throat and it can also result in the ulceration and tearing of the esophageal lining. Without correction this condition can become a serious health issue. The lining of the esophagus can be eroded by the presence of the stomach contents breaching through the esophageal valve, whose primary function is to prevent such occurrences. Most of the symptoms of acid-reflux can be prevented or dramatically reduced by means of proper daily hydration, proper chewing and attention to eating fewer acid-forming foods and drinking fewer acid-forming beverages (p 208).

- The stomach: The stomach is shaped like an elongated melon and has a valve on top and at the bottom. The esophageal valve is on top, and the pyloric valve or pyloric sphincter is at the bottom. These two valves are supposed to seal themselves shut and allow for a lot of rhythmical churning of the stomach contents, once we have finished swallowing all the food we plan to eat at any given meal or snack. The stomach is primarily responsible for digesting or breaking down protein. (Beef, chicken, fish, beans, legumes, etc.) Glands underneath the stomach mucosa (mucous lining) produce an enzyme called *protease* to break down protein.

- How much food can our stomach reasonably contain? This is a very important consideration. The normal size of any adult human stomach is about the size of your own clenched fist and possibly two fists. This means that for most people, they are eating way too much food at almost every meal, but particularly the evening meal. What this means is that their stomach is probably stretched bigger and larger than it should be. Practice eating an amount close to something comparable to one or two clenched fists. Practice eating an amount of food per meal that feels close to 75% full. It is very insulting to the stomach to eat to fullness. Many people eat beyond the full and normal capacity of their stomachs. This is the root cause of so many digestive problems. If you eat less and chew more, your stomach will slowly but surely return to its normal size and shape and function. Eat less, chew more.

- When we drink water, the water is able to be absorbed through the stomach lining and goes directly into our bloodstream and into our cells. Alcohol does the same thing. But almost all other liquids and foods remain in the stomach until they are passed on to the next stage of digestion. Too much liquid during a meal can dilute the effectiveness of the gastric juices secreted in the stomach. Hydrochloric acid is released in the stomach and has two primary purposes: to disinfect our food and to break down protein molecules into their individual amino acid components. The stomach has a thick mucous lining which serves as protection from the hydrochloric acid. If you are not properly hydrated, the mucous lining of your stomach may be too thin and this could cause many problems, including stomach ulcers. If you are not properly hydrated your stomach may not be able to produce enough hydrochloric acid. When this is the case, proteins will not be digested. Stomach contents will be released too soon. Undigested food particles will appear in the stool. Taking antacid tablets will not correct this problem and could make it worse. What corrects this problem is being properly hydrated, chewing food completely, and having full-spectrum micronutrients flowing into the bloodstream on a daily basis, along with supplemental digestive enzymes and probiotics. More on these things shortly.

- Food needs to remain in the stomach for one to three hours (or longer depending on *what* and *how much* was eaten). The lighter the meal, the less time required to churn. The more protein, the longer the churning. When protein is consumed, the stomach pumps out a large volume of hydrochloric acid. This drops the pH of the stomach in the neighborhood of 2.3, which is extremely acidic. When this happens, food will stay longer in the stomach. Slowly, the pH will rise. If the stomach contents are released too soon, you can invite a duodenal ulcer. (The duodenum requires a higher pH range for normal functioning.) The digestive system works its way back and forth between acid and alkaline states throughout the entire digestive system. Alkaline in the mouth, very acidic in the stomach; less acidic in the duodenum, small and large intestines. When you are hydrated, eat balanced properly prepared meals, chew well, and do not have micro-nutrient deficiencies, the proper pH balances are maintained automatically. This is another example of homeostasis.

- Under normal conditions, the stomach knows when the food it has been churning is ready to be released into the next phase of digestion. Generally speaking, this happens when the pH of the stomach contents rises to the appropriate level. One danger in taking any antacid or acid blocking medication is that it artificially and arbitrarily raises the pH level without regard to whether the food has been properly digested or not. The long-term use of stomach acid blocking medications eventually causes other digestive problems which can be worse than the original problem. The series of four valves in our digestive system are all connected: the esophageal valve, the pyloric valve, the ileo-cecal valve (which connects our small intestine to our large intestine), and the rectal valve or anal sphincter muscle. This last valve is the only one that is voluntary and within our control. Once the pyloric valve opens, emptying its contents into the duodenum, a signal is sent to the other remaining valves, and we will have the urge to eliminate (defecate). Under normal conditions, the urge to eliminate will be felt within one to three hours after the completion of any significant meal or snack. Imagine that.

- The duodenum: The duodenum is the first part of the small intestine. It receives the contents of digested food directly from the stomach. It also receives bile salts and other digestive enzymes from the gall bladder, which it gets from the liver and pancreas. These materials are designed to emulsify or break down fats in our diet. It is true that the gastric juices (also called pancreatic juices), contain digestive enzymes for the breaking down of carbohydrates, protein and fat. However, the strength and potency of these enzymes are directly proportional to our current state of health. Our current state of health is directly proportional to our levels of hydration-dehydration, nutrient deficiencies-toxic excess, intestinal dysbiosis, and general stress factors in the rest of our diet and lifestyle as previously described. If you are currently suffering from any kind of digestive system problem, you can safely and correctly assume that the relative strength and potency of the digestive enzymes in your pancreatic juices are not sufficient to produce normal digestion of your foods. Therefore, you need to pay attention to all the habits that facilitate normal digestion, including the use of supplemental digestive enzymes. We will discuss all of these things in Section Two.
- Carbohydrates are (primarily) digested in the mouth. Fiber foods may contain nutrients. All fiber foods must be properly chewed or they will not release their nutrients. Proteins get digested in the stomach. Fats get digested in the duodenum, which sits at the very top of the small intestine. Within a few inches the duodenum narrows to a tube about half an inch in diameter. The small intestine is 24 feet long.
- By the time our food reaches the first foot or two of the small intestine, it should be in a completely liquid state. This liquid slush of food is called chyme. Chyme travels into sections of the small intestine to begin the lengthy and important process of nutrient absorption. Each section is between 3-6 inches long. This is called segmentation. The gurgling sounds we often hear after meals is not always food churning around in the stomach, but could be coming from the rhythmic sloshing back and forth of our liquified food in the various segments of our small intestine.
- Billions, perhaps trillions of tiny finger-like projections appear along the wall of the small intestine. These projections are called villi. At the tip of each villi are smaller projections called micro-villi. The purpose of the villi and micro-villi is to identify certain nutrients in our food and extract them. These villi and micro-villi

function the very same way as do the roots of a plant in mineral-rich soil. As the roots of a plant suck nutrients from the soil, so the villi and micro-villi suck nutrients from our liquified food, passing these nutrients directly into our bloodstream. These blood vessels travel directly to the liver (via the hepatic or portal vein) for final inspection, selection (detoxification), and storage. What is not absorbed and assimilated into our bloodstream is passed on as waste and sent on to the large intestine.

- Providing direct assistance to the villi and micro-villi of the small intestine are trillions of microscopic beneficial bacteria. The dominant beneficial bacteria of the small intestine is called acidophilus. Beneficial bacteria, called probiotics, help to maintain the pH balances throughout the digestive system. Probiotics help in the absorption and assimilation of nutrients. Probiotics produce B vitamins and enzymes. Probiotics displace pathological bacteria. Probiotics produce their own antibiotics. Probiotics nourish and support the normal barrier function of the mucous lining that runs the length and breadth of the entire digestive system.

- Perhaps most importantly, the small intestine is home to specialized glands called Peyer's Patches (named after the scientist who discovered them). The Peyer's Patches are responsible for the production of about 80% of the antibody producing cells of the human immune system. These cells, like the natural killer cells, have the ability to identify and destroy foreign substances, abnormal cells and cancer cells. When the small intestines are functioning normally, the human immune system is functioning normally too. If the small intestines are not functioning normally, then the immune system is compromised, inviting the entire range of auto-immune disorders to take root and flourish; not just in the digestive system, but everywhere in the body.

- The small intestines twist and turn around like a bowl of spaghetti in water and occupy the area surrounding our belly-button or navel. Recall that in our mother's womb, we received nourishment from her uterus directly into our small intestine through the umbilical cord. Our belly-button or navel is a constant reminder of the physical source of our life. What our mothers ate and drank and were exposed to while we were in the womb has already determined a lot about who we are and how we have done so far in our lives, in terms of physical health. It is no small coincidence that our small intestine continues to be the root of our physical health.

Section 1 - Getting Ready

- At the end of the small intestine is a valve called the ileo-cecal valve. This valve is the intersection between the small intestine and the large intestine. The small intestine is called the ileum and the large intestine is called the cecum. On the large intestine side of this valve you find the vermiform appendix or just appendix. For years this was thought to be useless and was removed routinely, even if it was not infected or inflamed, as in appendicitis. However, Functional Medical doctors and researchers have discovered that the appendix secretes specialized chemicals to make sure that waste leaving the small intestine does not back up and go the wrong way. There are no parts of the human body that serve no function. There are simply parts and pieces of our anatomy and physiology that we don't understand yet. Rather than surgically removing them, we ought to nourish and protect them. No doubt in the future we will discover just how important all the pieces really are. Though no

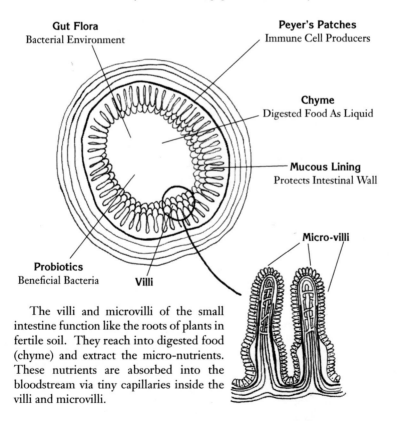

Cross Section of the Small Intestine
(duodenum, jejunum, ileum)

Gut Flora — Bacterial Environment
Peyer's Patches — Immune Cell Producers
Chyme — Digested Food As Liquid
Mucous Lining — Protects Intestinal Wall
Micro-villi
Probiotics — Beneficial Bacteria
Villi

The villi and microvilli of the small intestine function like the roots of plants in fertile soil. They reach into digested food (chyme) and extract the micro-nutrients. These nutrients are absorbed into the bloodstream via tiny capillaries inside the villi and microvilli.

parts of our anatomy and physiology are expendable, it is amazing nevertheless to observe how the body is able to compensate and continue to function after illness, injury, or removal of certain internal organs or parts of them.

- As digested food enters the large intestine, it is mostly waste and water. In the first several feet of large intestine (called the ascending colon), which is located on the right side of the abdomen, excess water is reabsorbed into the body and the remaining material starts to take on the texture and shape of fecal waste. This is toxic material that must be eliminated from the body in a timely manner. This means that from the time waste first enters the large intestine until it is eliminated into your toilet bowl (colon transit time), should be around 12 hours. Total transit time for any normal-sized meal should be right around 24 hours. This means the time it takes to travel the entire length of the digestive system, from mouth to stomach to toilet bowl. Too much shorter than this and you may not be absorbing nutrients effectively. Too much longer than this qualifies as a sluggish bowel or even constipation.

The Normal Colon

colon is the term used to refer to the large intestine

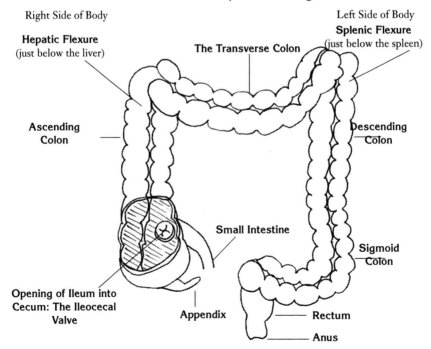

Section 1 - Getting Ready

- The problem with a sluggish bowel is that the large intestine or colon presses on or touches almost every major organ inside the human body, except the brain. Whether in proximity or actually touching, the risk of impairment to normal functioning of all these other internal organs is very great indeed. It is a question worth examining why prostate cancers in men and cervical and uterine cancers in women, are so high. These organs are in direct contact with the descending colon (called the sigmoid colon) and rectum. If waste is backed up and remains too long inside the body, common sense tells us that bad things might happen as a result. Who wants to live next door to a toxic waste site?

- The proper functioning of the large intestine or colon will turn out to be one of the key pieces of the puzzle, not just of digestive system health, but of the health of every other organ, system and cell in the entire body. We need to keep our colon clean!

- We have two feet of ascending colon on the right side and two feet of transverse colon which crosses right to left, from liver to spleen just below our rib cage and several inches above our navel. We

The Abnormal Colon

colon is the term used to refer to the large intestine

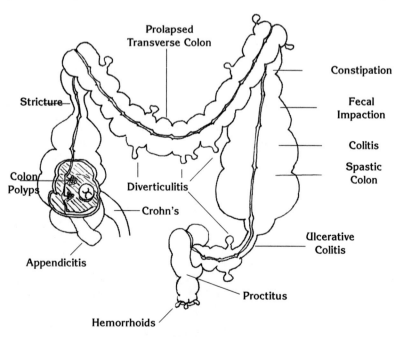

Healing Digestive Illness - **56**

have two feet of descending colon moving down the left side of our abdomen. It takes a sharp s-like curve near the pit of the abdominal area (this is called the sigmoid colon) and then enters the rectum which is the final waiting area for waste to be eliminated. Please keep in mind that the rectum is only about six inches long. Bowel movements can often be 12 to 18 inches long or longer. This means that the waste material is waiting inside the rectum and much of the sigmoid colon too. These organs directly press upon the prostate, bladder, pelvic girdle and sciatic nerve in men; and the vagina, cervix, bladder, uterus, ovaries, pelvic girdle, and sciatic nerve in women.

- Proper elimination of fecal waste is one of the most important functions of the digestive system. Examination and confirmation of a healthy bowel movement is one of the most important self-assessment tools we can develop and utilize every day. Ask any Naturalist worth her salt what's the easiest way to determine the health of any animal in the wild and they will tell you this: *Examine the scat.* Scat is what naturalists call fecal waste or the bowel movement of the animal. It is the same with us. If your bowel movements are regular, normal and consistently healthy (as defined below), you can sleep more easily knowing that one of the most important functions of your body is functioning the way it is supposed to. It is rare to find anyone with a perfectly functioning digestive and eliminative system, and also find serious health problems in other areas of the body. When the digestive and eliminative systems are functioning properly, everything else in our body benefits. In the next paragraphs let me share some more information I give to my clients in the first few days of their *Intestinal Regeneration Program.* This information describes the ideal bowel movement and provides instructions for figuring out your digestive transit time.

The Ideal Bowel Movement

While it is increasingly important, and sometimes downright urgent, for everyone to become more familiar with the inner workings of their own digestive systems, in particular the large intestine or colon, it is also important to keep our sense of humor and perspective. Many years ago when I was first learning about colon health, colon cleansing, and the importance of healthy pooping and transit time, I came across the term, Golden Banana, and it has stuck with me ever since. What is the Golden Banana? The Golden Banana refers to the shape and size, texture and color of the ideal bowel movement. (With sincere apologies to all banana lovers/consumers everywhere.)

Since the normal size of the adult human large intestine is five to six feet long and about two inches in diameter (inner diameter), we should be producing bowel movements that measure about two inches in diameter. The shape of the sigmoid colon, the last part of the colon before the rectum and anus, gives the bowel movement its characteristic curved shape, which to many can be compared favorably with the curves of a tropical banana.

The ideal bowel movement then, is two inches in diameter, but can be anywhere from six to nine to twelve inches in length, or more, depending upon the volume of food that has been consumed. Transit time (or the time it takes for a complete meal to travel the entire length of the digestive system from the mouth to the toilet bowl), must be within the 18-24 hour window for optimal health purposes. The texture of the bowel movement should be soft (like soft serve ice cream

Section 1 - Getting Ready

or creamy peanut butter), and it should come out easily, effortlessly, without straining or pushing, grunting or groaning. It should only take several seconds or at most a minute or two to empty one's bowels. The color should be light brown, not dark brown, not black, and certainly not green or white or any other color, although some discoloration can occur depending on the foods eaten. Beets will turn the feces reddish. Too many carrots will turn the feces orange. Too much meat and cheese, and foods combining butter, sugar, and flour will turn the feces black and hard and heavy and dry and slow.

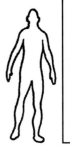

The length of the entire human digestive system is approximately thirty feet long, from mouth to anus. This is five times the length of a person measuring six feet tall.

Checking Our Transit Time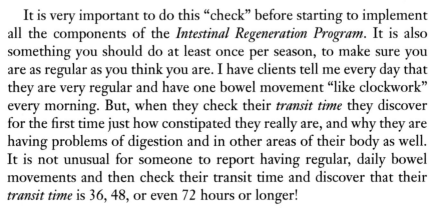

It is very important to do this "check" before starting to implement all the components of the *Intestinal Regeneration Program*. It is also something you should do at least once per season, to make sure you are as regular as you think you are. I have clients tell me every day that they are very regular and have one bowel movement "like clockwork" every morning. But, when they check their *transit time* they discover for the first time just how constipated they really are, and why they are having problems of digestion and in other areas of their body as well. It is not unusual for someone to report having regular, daily bowel movements and then check their transit time and discover that their *transit time* is 36, 48, or even 72 hours or longer!

Here is a very easy way to check your transit time. Go to the supermarket and purchase three or four medium sized organic red beets. (Yes, if you can't get organic, just use the regular beets.) Wash them, cut them up, then steam them or boil them until they are ready to eat. Chew thoroughly. You can do this separately, or alongside any meal. Take note of the time you finished eating the beets. You will probably notice the effect of the red beets in your urine before you see them in your bowel movements. Be prepared to have a reddish discoloration of your urine. This is not blood. It's the beets. Look for the color of your next bowel movement to be dark brown or reddish brown. I once had a client tell me that the color of their bowel movement was the color of the Crayola crayon *Burnt Siena*. Take note of the time the red beets show up mixed in with your bowel movement and end up in the toilet bowl. This will give you your transit time.

Section 1 - Getting Ready

One should feel "complete" when the bowel movement has exited the body. There should be no sensation that there is still more fecal matter, up there, unwilling to come out. One should not have to wipe excessively. One should feel relieved and at peace for doing one's duty. One should feel eager to exclaim: *All is right with the world; I have just produced another golden banana!*

The frequency of our bowel movements is a topic of considerable importance. I talk to people every day who only have one or two bowel movements per week, during a good week. But the real tragedy is that they have been told by their doctors (or others) that this is normal. This has become common, but I can assure you that it is not normal. What's normal is to have at least one or two bowel movements per day. What's normal is to completely eliminate from your body all the foods and beverages you consumed within the previous 24 hour period. If this is not happening then you run the risk of *toxemia* or self-poisoning from the osmotic seepage of fecal waste through the colon walls into the bloodstream. (This is a form of leaky gut syndrome.) This is a very real danger. Ideal frequency is to have a bowel movement within one hour of any significant meal or snack. This is the way the digestive system is designed to function. Check your personal transit time on a regular basis, at least once per season.

Remember our tour of the digestive system earlier? Remember the series of valves at the various locations along the way? These valves are all connected and are communicating with each other all the time. At least they are supposed to be communicating. The esophageal valve lets food into the stomach. The pyloric valve lets food into the duodenum, which is the beginning of the small intestine. The ileo-cecal valve lets food (now waste) into the cecum or large intestine, and the last valve in our series is the only one containing voluntary muscles, making it mostly within our total control; the anal sphincter. If you allow a normal amount of time between meals, say three or four hours, you can see that each major meal will have exited the stomach at the time the next meal is due to arrive. Given any normal 24 hour period, there will be three or four meals at various stages and locations inside the digestive system: stomach, small intestines, large intestine, and sigmoid colon most especially. As each new meal leaves the stomach, messages are sent to the other corresponding valves, signaling them to release their contents into the next section/stage of digestion. This is how our digestive system, *our primary elimination system*, is designed to function. So you can see that ideally, the frequency of our bowel movements is connected to the number of meals we have daily.

Section 1 - Getting Ready

This is as good a time as any to acknowledge some of the masters of colon health of the last century: John Harvey Kellogg, Weston Price, Bernard Jensen, John Anderson among many illustrious and colorful *others*. Check out the *Resources* section for their book titles. One of our current-day masters of colon health education is Dr. Richard Schulze, who runs the American Botanical Pharmacy in Marina del Rey, California. Here's what he has to say about the ideal frequency of our bowel movements:

> Primitive peoples living in remote non-industrialized regions of the world as recently as fifty years ago were discovered to average about 2 to 4 bowel movements per day. These relaxed primitive people all seemed to have one bowel movement within 20 or 30 minutes after each major meal. They would just squat, stuff would come out, and within a minute they were done. No library of magazines, no squeezing, straining, grunting, moaning, meditation, or prayer. It would just come out effortlessly. These people averaged between 2 and 4 bowel movements a day or 14 to 28 bowel movements per week. When we compare this to the typical constipated American bowel habit of one bowel movement every 3 to 5 days or 2 or 3 bowel movements per week, the comparison is shocking. I figure this comparison puts the average American about 70,000 bowel movements short in their lifetime! (Dr. Richard Schulze, *Healing Colon Disease Naturally* [Santa Monica: CA Natural Healing Publications, 1999], 36)

Remembering the ideal posture for the very best elimination of waste is also a very important consideration. To get a sense of what proper fecal elimination feels like, try either to remember a time or imagine a time when you were out in a forest, alone, exploring; and suddenly you had that unmistakable urge to have a bowel movement. First you had to find the right tree, preferably on a slight slope. You pulled down your pants and then grabbed the tree, positioning yourself on the downside slope. You gently squatted down bending from the knees, still hanging onto the tree with both hands. The laws of gravity take over from here resulting in the easy, smooth, effortless elimination of a golden banana-like bowel movement.

Section 1 - Getting Ready

If you can approximate this experience on your own toilet bowl at home fantastic. Otherwise you may need to look into how you can. It could be as easy as positioning a few wooden blocks under each foot as you sit down. There are companies who make such products, and companies pioneering new kinds of toilet bowls to accommodate this traditional information about the ideal posture required to have a safe, comfortable, relaxed, and effective bowel movement. Like the first three rules of yoga, our bowel movements should be similarly defined: relax, breathe and never strain.

The Great American Pastime

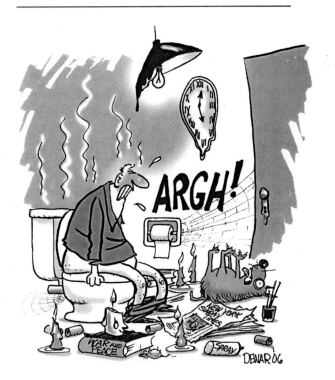

As usual, George has run out of reading material.

Section 1 - Getting Ready

The Power of True Stories

> *The Universe is made up of stories, not atoms.*
> Muriel Rukeyser, Poet

Never underestimate the power of true stories of individual personal healing to inspire you to make the decision to take the consistent actions that will produce the results you want in your life. These actions and decisions will be the things that nourish you best.

The stories in this book are from people I have worked with directly using the exact same information, recipes, supplements and other products that I am suggesting to you. It worked for me. It worked for them. It will work for you too. Just don't take any short-cuts or make any compromises or leave anything out. Don't make the mistake of thinking that you can substitute this for that and get the same results. I can only promise you results if you use the same information, recipes, products and services that I use and recommend in my practice and in this book. Every aspect of this *Intestinal Regeneration Program* has been discovered, worked on and mastered to a very significant degree over a long and rigorous forty-year period. It ain't broke, so don't try to fix it. It works!

Over the years I have come to know many professional storytellers, people who tell folk tales and fairy tales, at libraries, in schools and in concert. These folks tell their stories from memory because they have learned them *by heart* in the ancient ways of the oral tradition. When you are first learning a story, you need to really stick to the exact details of the story as it first comes to you. That's called *honoring the*

Section 1 - Getting Ready

muse, honoring the tradition, honoring the source of the story. Later on, once you have gained a certain mastery of the materials inside the story, you are granted certain liberties and one of those liberties is to alter or change the materials inside the story. This is how new stories are created. This is how the oldest stories make their way into the present time. Storytellers may change the clothes of the story, but the heart and soul of the story remains the same down through the ages. And these *true stories* continue to nourish us every single day.

My point is a simple one. Learn the fundamentals of Functional Nutrition as they are explained in my *Intestinal Regeneration Program* in this book.

Once you have mastered these fundamentals, you should feel absolutely free to change anything you want, change as much as you want and ultimately make it into your own program. Not only do I encourage you to do this, I want you to do this. *But do not put the cart before the horse.* Just take one step at a time. Learn and master the fundamentals of this program before you start looking for ways to make any changes or improvements. This will take at least several months to a year of due diligence on your part. Then, after this time has passed, if you believe you have made some important discoveries and made some improvements to the program, by all means contact me and let me know.

Note from RM: As I work on the second edition of Healing Digestive Illness, I think it is important to point out that even though many thousands of people have read the above paragraph, not one person in the eight years since the original publication of this book in 2006 has contacted me to announce an improvement to the program. Three years ago, I was introduced to the new science of Redox Biochemistry. Discoveries being made in this science will be reflected in my future books and ebooks. If you would like to learn more about Redox Biochemistry and how it can improve your digestive wellness you can contact me through my website: russellmariani@healingdigestiveillness.com

Simply keep in mind that this program is the result of forty years of constant study and experimentation of my own and the direct experience of thousands of my seminar participants and clients. So please be patient and plan on mastering the fundamentals first as described in this book.

There are some people in the world, and I am one of them, who believe strongly in the healing power of the oral tradition. This oral tradition includes stories and songs, ballads and poems. Some are works of pure fiction; some are based on real occurrences. Some are myths and some are legends and some are total fabrications and out and out lies. But almost all stories, if told from the heart of the storyteller, contain some relevant and important kernels of truth. And this truth can speak to the heart of the listener in ways that bypass all logic and reasoning. This experience is true not only of the creative and expressive arts, but of the healing arts as well. We gain insight into the root causes of our own problems and our own solutions by paying more attention to our own story and the stories of others. As one of my first successful clients once revealed to me, *"I have learned to listen to my body and honor what I hear."*

These truths, often found in the oddest and most unlikely of places and circumstances can motivate and inspire and transform the reader or listener or participant. Let me give you an example from my own life.

In the spring of 1977, I was a senior in college and already four full years into my journey to better health through better nutritional choices but I was feeling completely lost and all alone. I had made some progress, but most of the books I read caused me greater confusion not less. Most of the seminars I took piled on more misinformation not less. Most of the doctors and therapists I spoke with increased my level of uncertainty they didn't decrease it.

I had a *growing inner knowing* that my body was a sacred temple that I needed to take better care of, but the literature in nutrition was all chemical, mathematical, analytical. I once asked a *nutrition expert*, a Registered Dietician, how sugar affects the body and she proceeded to draw on a piece of paper the chemical breakdown of carbon atoms to glucose to water. This explanation was not helpful to me at all. I was losing hope. I was an English major and a Philosophy minor. I needed these things explained to me in plain language. I needed something different than the mainstream approach. I needed a mere molecule of hope. I needed some evidence that I was on the right path in my pursuit of better health through better nutrition. That molecule of hope appeared one night at a poetry reading on the campus of Rutgers University in New Brunswick, New Jersey.

The poet was Robert Bly. Perhaps some of you have heard of him, read his books, or even better had the opportunity to hear him "live." Robert is a master of the oral tradition and that night back in 1977 was my very first experience of the healing power of the spoken arts. Bly never once opened a book during his entire three hour performance. How can I explain this? There was a truth that I was searching for, and a truth that he was somehow able to embody in the way he spoke his stories and read his poems. He didn't explain or reveal any truth in any straightforward or logical way. He didn't say: *Olympia is the capital of Washington*. It was a *metaphorical truth* that I was seeing and hearing and feeling. A perennial truth about the human condition itself. A truth that had been true for a thousand years. A truth that was buried in my own heart, mind and soul. A truth that slowly started to reveal itself to me during the course of the poetry reading that night. A truth that rang out loud and clear in the middle of one particular poem.

> *Inside this clay jug there are canyons and pine mountains,*
> *and the maker of canyons and pine mountains!*
>
> *All seven oceans are inside, and hundreds of millions of stars.*
> *The acid that tests gold is there, and the one who judges jewels.*
> *And the music from the strings no one touches, and the*
> *source of all water.*
>
> *If you want the truth, I will tell you the truth:*
> *Friend, listen: the God whom I love is inside.*

Sufi poet Kabir, translated by Robert Bly.
The Kabir Book, [Boston, Beacon Press, 1971]

    A truth found its way into the center of my existence that night and I have never understood the world the same way since. This truth is that true personal healing will be found in the proper care and maintenance of the cells of the human body. This truth is that the greatest of all human needs is the need to take care of our cells and the cells of those we love. This truth is that we are all the children of one creation and one God. This truth is that we are all brothers and sisters in one human family and that we are here together at this time in history to learn the hard lessons of loving the earth and each other with vision and compassion, wisdom and justice, for the purpose of personal and planetary peace. This truth is that we are all here to learn about and do the things that nourish us best.

    Never underestimate the power of true stories of individual personal healing to inspire you to make the decision to take the consistent actions that will produce the results you want in your life. These actions and decisions will be the things that nourish you best.

    Once you are well and you truly believe that you have mastered the fundamentals of functional nutrition described in this book, please feel free to experiment like crazy. But right now, for *your* best results, just follow the bouncing ball of each and every suggestion in this book.

Section 1 - Getting Ready

Stay true to the heart of the healing stories I am about to share with you, and chances are that your own story will end up being happily ever after too.

A good story speaks to the heart of the listener.
A good storyteller speaks from the heart of the story.
Megan Moore, Storyteller.

Section 1 - Getting Ready

🌰 Russell's Story: Ulcerative Colitis, Anxiety, Depression

I had been sick for about a year but the seriousness of my symptoms never registered: constipation for days at a time, then diarrhea for days at a time. I lived on Kaopectate and Pepto Bismol depending on my condition and symptoms. I was uncomfortable all the time. I had constant headaches and my face was a mess with acne. I was tired all the time. I felt lousy. I had constant indigestion, constant gas and bloating, constant abdominal discomfort and episodes of acute abdominal pain. I had intestinal cramps that were so bad, that they literally threw me out of my bed in the middle of night. I would curl up in a fetal position on the floor of my bedroom and moan for hours. I never had a good night's sleep. I probably had insomnia. I remember lying awake for hours every night. I never had a normal bowel movement. Ropey little stringy things, or hard round black balls, or one variation or other or loose bowel movements right up to full blown diarrhea. I never told anyone about any of this. I was too embarrassed. I was too ashamed. It was late winter, 1973. I had just turned 18 years old.

Months and months had gone by and nothing seemed to change. Then one night something really weird happened. I sat up in bed feeling the unstoppable urgency that had defined my regular bouts of diarrhea. I ran to the bathroom and made it just in the nick of time, as usual. It sounded like normal diarrhea, but as I turned around to flush, I was shocked to discover that the toilet bowl was filled with bright red blood. My blood.

I was very freaked out.

The next day proved to be even stranger. My appointment with the gastro-enterologist was scheduled for 11 am. The waiting room

Section 1 - Getting Ready

was filled with older men. No one in the room was under 60 years of age, except me. Remember that this was 1973. Men looked older at younger ages back then. The difference between the generations was more pronounced back then. Many things were different back then. By three pm the waiting room was empty. The nurse came out and asked me who I was and why I was sitting there. I told her my name and said that my appointment was for 11 am. The nurse explained that the doctor never saw patients my age and that she assumed I was the son or grandson of one of the other patients. Then she explained that the reason the doctor never saw patients my age was because the kind of problems the doctor treated didn't usually happen to people until they turned 50 or older. I am sure she was trying to be reassuring, but it made me feel even more strange and isolated than before. She apologized for keeping me waiting all day and brought me in to see the doctor.

I endured the excruciating pain and absolute humiliation of a full-length colonoscopy without any anesthesia. It wasn't even an option back then. (Well, it wasn't offered to me anyway.) Once the procedure started, there was nothing I could do. I felt trapped. I couldn't believe the level of discomfort and pain I was experiencing! I screamed out every curse word and unsavory phrase I could think of. I didn't even know who this doctor was, but I decided that I hated him. I couldn't wait to get out of there, and was determined to walk out just as soon as I could. Finally, "the procedure" was over. I couldn't believe I had just willingly submitted myself to such a horrendous experience. I started looking for the door. I wasn't interested in talking to anyone. I wanted to get the hell out of there.

Halfway to the door, the doctor grabbed me by the arm. "Son, you just can't walk out of here like that. Besides I have some bad news for you. You need to sit down for this."

"Sit down?" I thought to myself, "I may not be able to sit down for a week after what I just went through!" Once again, I felt like I had no choice. I reluctantly and cautiously sat down inside the austere confines of that ill-fated examination room in the middle of what was shaping up to be one of the worst days of my life. Unbelievably, it got worse.

"It looks like you have colon cancer." The doctor had just spoken. "We have to run some more tests, but it does not look good." I'm sure he said a lot more than that, but that is all I remember. My mind was spinning in a million different directions. Cancer? How is that possible? Cancer? People die from cancer! Cancer? Me? I'm too young to have cancer! Cancer? I was totally shocked. I had never been in a situation like this before. I felt totally helpless and alone. I was terrified.

What seemed like an eternity probably lasted only thirty seconds. The doctor was waiting for my response and I was trying to come up with one.

Instinctively, my mind was racing around for an explanation, a reason, an excuse, a justification, anything. Suddenly, I had a question to ask:

"Do you think this has anything to do with my diet?"

His answer, as it turned out, changed my life.

"No." he said. "There's no connection."

"Well then, what causes colon cancer?" I asked.

"We don't know. (he paused) Stress."

Then he left it at that and left the room.

Stress? I had never experienced so much stress in my entire life! I left the doctors office that afternoon determined to find out how and why I had gotten myself into such a mess. In spite of my doctor's assurances that "more tests were needed" before they knew *for sure* what was wrong with me, I was already gearing up for the worst case scenario. I was also starting to feel that I might have to start figuring things out on my own. By the time I got home that night, I had the very distinct and very disquieting feeling that I was definitely going to *have to* figure things out on my own.

Why did I ask my doctor the question about diet? It was *not* because I knew anything about the connections between diet and disease, nutrition, and health; because at that time in my life, I didn't. I asked the question because it was the only thing that made sense. You see, since the previous summer, I had been on a high-protein diet, where I ate steak three times a day, and as much milk and cheese and ice cream as I wanted. I had never connected my many uncomfortable gastro-intestinal symptoms to my high-protein diet, until that moment. I can't tell you how or why I knew there was a connection between my symptoms and my diet. But I can tell you this: ***I knew there was a connection***!

The doctor said there was no connection between my diet and my condition, but I believed there was. The doctor said they didn't know what caused colon cancer, other than stress. I certainly didn't know for sure what had caused my condition and symptoms. I only knew that the answer; "We don't know" didn't make any sense at all. This was America! Land of the free, home of the brave! This was America! We were landing men on the moon! We had the very best medicine on earth! Or so I had been lead to believe. Surely we could figure out the cause and cure for colon cancer. I was determined to find out what caused my condition and symptoms. I was determined to find a cure and get better fast. I had no choice. I had to find a cure. I was too young to die!

(Please remember that I was looking for a "cure" because I was just starting out on my journey. At this point in time I did not know the difference between curing and personal healing as I described earlier.)

In the three weeks between my first examination and my next series of tests, I went to the library almost every day looking up whatever literature I could find about the connections between diet and colon cancer. Here's what I discovered:

The lack of fiber in the diet has been identified as a major contributing factor in an increasingly higher and higher rate of colon cancer in both men and women.

I can't tell you from what book or study or author I read the above sentence. I simply can't remember and I never wrote down the exact quotation or source. All I can tell you is that when I read these words (or something like them), I knew instantly that I had found the first clue in solving the puzzle of my own personal health crisis. I was ecstatic. I was relieved. I was hopeful once again. I was looking forward to sharing my discovery with my doctor. My next encounter with my doctor turned about to be another interesting experience.

He laughed at me. When I told my doctor what I had discovered about the link between dietary fiber and colon cancer, he laughed at me! He said there was no connection. He looked at me with an expression combining disgust and pity, as if I were the biggest fool alive. Then he lowered the boom: "Besides" he said with some measure of relief in his voice, "You don't have colon cancer. Not yet anyway. But don't get me wrong, your colon is a mess. You have a very serious case of pre-cancerous ulcerative colitis." He went on and on but I stopped listening after the first few sentences.

I remember thinking to myself that I was supposed to meet this news about my ulcerative colitis as if it were *good news*, as if this was better than colon cancer, which it was, technically, but somehow it just didn't feel that way. There was very little *good news* in any of this for me at the time. I just felt angry and confused and humiliated. In spite of all the feelings swirling around inside of me that afternoon, I felt pretty certain about three things when I left his office:

I did not like this doctor.

I did not trust this doctor.

If I was going to get better, I was going to have to do it on my own.

It never entered my mind to seek a second or third opinion. Imagine that.

In the days and weeks following my informative encounters with the *gastroenterologist*, I read a series of books that I had found about the connections between diet and disease. I'm pretty sure that one of those books was entitled: *Are You Confused?* written by the famous Naturopathic doctor, Paavo Airola. I took the book off the shelf because I most certainly was confused. I read a few chapters and felt more confused. I read another book called: *The Save Your Life Diet*, written by Dr. David Reuben. I took this book off the shelf because the title really spoke to me. Literally. The basic premise of David Reuben's book was that colon cancer was caused by too much meat and dairy and processed foods and not enough fiber from whole foods like grains, fruits, and vegetables. His book made a lot of sense to me.

I took myself off the crazy high protein diet right away. I dramatically decreased the amount of meat, dairy and processed foods in my diet. I dramatically increased the amount of fiber in my diet. I think the first month on my "new diet" I ate three bowls of bran cereal every single day. I ate salads and carrots and apples and bananas. My family and friends thought I had gone a little "nuts." I didn't care. I was on a mission. I was on a quest. In a matter of a few days, I started to feel and see results. In a matter of a few weeks, most of my physical symptoms were completely gone. What a revelation. What a sense of relief I felt. (I am not suggesting that you eat bran cereal. Please be patient. My complete dietary recommendations are in Section Two.)

Although my *physical symptoms* had cleared up rather quickly, my emotional, mental or psychological symptoms did not. The months of constant digestive problems had taken their toll. The weeks of absolute terror I lived through believing that I had colon cancer and might die as a result, *with the best doctors in the world not knowing the cause or the cure*, left me anxious, uncertain and afraid. Though some pieces of the diet and health puzzle made sense to me, many other pieces remained elusive. The more I read, the more confused I became. The more "diets" I tried, the more frustrated I became. No matter how hard I tried, I never really felt 100% healthy again, the way I had felt before the onset of all my digestive system problems, sometime in the Spring of 1972.

The worst symptoms I endured as an aftermath of all my experiences with ulcerative colitis, modern medicine and the hundreds of conflicting choices available to me in the holistic and alternative healing worlds between 1973 and 1980 were these: anxiety and depression.

Sometimes these "states" of anxiety and depression would come upon me slowly and gradually. Sometimes they would hit me like a ton of bricks. Whenever they happened, they were always unwelcome guests. In the previous eighteen years of my life, I had never felt any anxiety or depression. I had always felt lots of good energy. I had always been enthusiastic and optimistic. I had always felt confident and successful. I hated feeling anxious and afraid. It felt like something from my personality had been stolen. These states of anxiety and depression always felt so foreign and strange. At my worst moments, I felt totally helpless and hopeless. At my worst moments I desperately feared for my life. At my worst moments I could feel parts of my personality slipping away, eroding away, disappearing and dissolving into some dark abyss, like an Edgar Allan Poe horror story that had become real. (My favorite writer as a high school student.)

During one of these darkest of times, an interesting realization occurred to me. "Perhaps there is some reason for my suffering." What that reason could be I could only begin to imagine, and what I imagined was usually not very favorable! And so I began to pray. I began to bargain with God. Here was the essence of my prayer: "Dear God! I hate feeling anxious and depressed. I hate feeling alone and isolated. I hate feeling adrift at sea, with no rudder, oars, sail, map, or compass. I hate feeling uncertain about the purpose and direction of my life. I know I am on the right path by changing my diet and lifestyle. I know I am on the right path to learn about the things that nourish me best. Here is my promise to you. If I can ever wake up in the morning once again, free of these awful feelings of uncertainty, anxiety and depression, I will dedicate the rest of my life to teaching others about the things that got me well and kept me well. I will dedicate the rest of my life to helping other people who are suffering the way I am suffering now. Please show me the way back to health and confidence, energy, vitality, and fun."

Section 1 - Getting Ready

During the years between 1973 and 1980, I read hundreds of books, joined many interesting organizations, attended dozens of seminars, and interviewed many experts about alternative health and healing. I experienced everything that was out there at the time, from Alcoholics Anonymous to Macrobiotics to Zen. I had jobs that exposed me to every aspect of the food and nutrition industries, from organic gardening to lab testing the seeds and nuts at the Erewhon Natural Foods Warehouse. I washed dishes and waited on tables and worked my way from vegetable cutter to head chef. I practiced meditation and yoga and learned many forms of bodywork and massage. I met thousands of people just like me, searching for the answers about the causes of their sickness and disease. I met thousands of people searching for solutions, searching for answers, searching for health. I met many people who healed themselves from cancer and other serious illnesses. I met many people who did not heal themselves as well. I witnessed many people who died from their illnesses at far too young an age. I learned important life-changing lessons from them all.

During the years between 1980 and 1987 I felt pretty good most of the time. But I never felt 100% healthy and energetic. My best days were about 80%. I figured that's just the way it's going to be. I was convinced I was doing the best that I could do and had already tried everything that was out there to try in the holistic and alternative world. I had a part-time practice in Shiatsu Massage and Nutrition Counseling. My dietary suggestions were often too extreme for other people to follow for any length of time, which was an endless source of frustration for me. I knew that people could heal themselves by eating certain foods and avoiding other foods, but most people were just not willing to make too many changes. People wanted magic bullet/quick fix solutions and I didn't have any to offer.

In the Spring of 1987, I was introduced to an amazing wild-crafted food called Super Blue Green Algae. I remember my first *algae experience* like it was yesterday. About two weeks after eating only two capsules of the algae per day, I woke up very early one morning and felt something very pleasant but also very strange. I felt 100% healthy and alive! I was sitting at my desk, and I remember looking at my legs and arms as if I could see the pulsation of my life-force coursing through my veins like some kind of visible electric current. I remember thinking to myself: Wow, this is unbelievable. This is how I used to feel when I was a teenager, before I got sick. I walked downstairs into our kitchen to see if Megan (my wife) was feeling the same thing.

Section 1 - Getting Ready

Our eyes met with the unmistakable expression: "Are you feeling what I'm feeling?" The answer was a resounding yes. The intensity of the experience wore off by the end of the day, but each day I continued to eat my algae, and every day I felt 100% healthy and alive again. What on earth was going on?

All I can tell you is this: based on everything I have studied before and since that time, there is only one logical explanation. Prior to the day that Super Blue Green Algae entered my life (and my bloodstream) I was suffering from micro-nutrient deficiencies. (This is one of the root causes for all physical degeneration and disease as I described earlier.) The algae contains over 80 different micro-nutrients from every significant category. The algae contains every vitamin except vitamin D, which we get from sunlight. The algae contains over 43 minerals and trace minerals. The algae contains active enzymes. The algae has the greatest amount of chlorophyll gram per gram than any other food. And chlorophyll is a cell builder and blood purifier. A molecule of chlorophyll and a molecule of hemoglobin (red blood cells) are identical in almost every way, except for an atom of iron which gives hemoglobin its red color and magnesium which gives chlorophyll its green color. Chlorophyll carries oxygen to the cells of our body.

The algae is the biggest source of beta-carotene, a powerful antioxidant. The algae contains all 20 amino acids, which is unique to all plants, and amino acids are the building blocks of protein. The physical structure of all cells is protein. Most of our human structure is made of protein. The algae contains complete protein molecules. This means that the basic building blocks are present in the algae for the cells of our body to do essential repair work; reconstruction, deconstruction, and new construction! The algae contains nucleic acids which provide vital nourishment for the inner machinery of all cells. The algae contains essential fatty acids like Omega 3 and Omega 6. And the algae contains all of these essential micro-nutrients in a form that is 100% digestible and easy to assimilate.

The body exerts no energy to get at these nutrients and there is no fiber and no waste. This Super Blue Green Algae is the most amazing single food source of vital nutrients that I have ever experienced and I have tried them all!

In the years between 1987 and 1994, I was mostly symptom free. I had no digestive system problems and the few moments of anxiety and depression were rare and mild.

In the Spring of 1994, I started to give seminars around the United States and Canada about the fundamentals of nutrition and health. I felt fantastic most of the time, but gradually the jet-setting lifestyle started to wear me out. In November of 1994, I was taken to the hospital after suffering my very first kidney stone attack. Unfortunately, it wasn't my last. It was the worst physical pain I had ever felt. After a few shots of morphine (in the hospital) to relax all my muscles, I passed the kidney stone the following morning.

After that unsettling experience, I started to have relapses with my old friends, anxiety and depression. I just could not imagine what was causing these symptoms to return. But return they did, with a vengeance. I examined every aspect of my diet and lifestyle and redoubled all my efforts in avoiding insulting foods and habits and stayed totally focused on complementary foods, beverages, supplements and other influences. In the summer of 1995, I passed another kidney stone. In October of 1996, I passed my third kidney stone in three years. I knew that if I didn't figure something out soon I would be heading straight towards the creation of my fourth kidney stone or something even worse. But I was distracted. My anxiety was becoming more frequent and near constant. I was starting to have extreme panic attacks. The only solution was to lock myself in my room and just wait it out. Depression was hovering around me constantly now, and the worst thing about all this was that I couldn't tell any one. I was Mr. Health Educator! I was Mr. Nutrition Counselor! I was used to figuring these things out and solving them alone.

In January 1997, for no apparent reason, I felt completely fine. The fog of depression had finally lifted and the constant panic attacks had stopped. As much as I enjoyed every precious moment of my reprieve, I couldn't help but thinking that another episode was just lurking around the corner. Now, trust me, I wanted desperately to think positive thoughts, but the truth was that I knew with confidence that I had absolutely no idea why my anxiety and depression had suddenly disappeared. This realization troubled me. And of course I still hadn't figured out what was causing them to appear in the first place. This was most troubling. I had learned so much about the puzzle of nutrition and health, but clearly a piece was still missing. I kept reading. I kept talking to my colleagues. I kept experimenting with my diet, modifying my lifestyle, but nothing seemed to help at all. Still, I was very grateful for my unexpected reprieve. I never knew how temporary these reprieves would ever be.

Then in February 1997, I flew down to Tampa, Florida from Boston to give one of my seminars. I remember walking on the beach on a Friday afternoon soon after my arrival. Clear blue skies, 80 degrees and

Section 1 - Getting Ready

brilliant sunshine. As I walked along the beach I remember thinking: Man do I feel great or what! This is just perfect. I wish I could bottle this moment and remember how to feel this way no matter what happens in the future. There were beach volley-ball games happening every 100 yards or so and I was thinking I would go and join one. Then, it hit me. Wham. Just like that. The lights went out again. The dimmer switch got turned all the way down. The air went out of my lungs. The darkness and shadows descended upon me. Fear roiled in the pit of my stomach. Depression. Just like that. I walked back to my hotel in shock and disbelief. In a few short hours, my seminar was set to begin. How was I going to pull it off this time?

Somehow, I survived. I always managed to survive. I kept on trusting and hoping and believing that there was an organic explanation for my suffering, even though I could not seem to find the right book or the right person to explain it to me. Not yet anyway. I just never stopped believing that the explanation was out there, somewhere. My job was to keep looking for it and never give up. Perhaps you know the feeling.

The following weekend I was in Tulsa, Oklahoma to give another one of my day-long seminars. I was half-way through the Saturday morning session, when a very troubling and distracting realization entered my mind: *You may never find the solution because you keep looking in all the wrong places.* Whoa. That thought really messed me up. I stopped lecturing. I remember looking out to a sea of puzzled and concerned faces. Beads of sweat broke out around the edges of my forehead. My mouth got really, really dry. I thought for sure I was going to melt-down right in front of everybody. Suddenly, I had an idea: "Folks," I said with a forced but passable smile on my face, "I sure hope you understand, but sometimes these things just happen. I've given this seminar a hundred times over the past few years and I can give this particular talk in my sleep forwards and backwards. But, I just had an unmistakable *brain cramp* and I've completely lost the thread of what I have been talking about." Everybody laughed. That helped. "Let's take an early lunch break. Let's get back together at one pm." It worked. Everyone got up and filed out of the room without incident. I turned around and shuffled through some papers on the lectern, trying to look unavailable and distracted and busy.

When I turned around to leave the room there was a strange looking man standing there waiting for me. He was skinny and disheveled, wearing denim overalls and a yellow plaid cotton shirt. He wore a scraggly day-old beard and was missing a front tooth or two. I didn't say a word to him. I just stared. He spoke first. "I was wondering if you have ever come across the connection between hydration and depression?" Say What? I thought I was hallucinating. Maybe I *had* melted down after all. Maybe everyone was still in the room. Maybe this man was a shamanic guide from the Carlos Castaneda books I had read in the early seventies. Before I could formulate a response to him, he started speaking again: "I think you need to read this book. Here, take it. It's a gift." He handed me the book, and I said thank you. Then he turned and walked away.

I stared down at the book cover and read the title to myself: *Your Body's Many Cries for Water*. And the subtitle, right below it: "You are not sick, you are thirsty!" By F. Batmanghelidj, MD. I tucked the book in my bag and walked to my room. I sat down on the side of my newly made bed and read through the table of contents, I scrolled my finger down to chapter five, *Stress and Depression*: the initially silent compensation mechanisms associated with dehydration. I turned to chapter five and started reading:

> A state of depression is said to exist when the brain, in confronting a stressful emotional problem finds it difficult to cope with other attention-demanding actions at the same time. This phenomenon can become so all-absorbing as to incapacitate the person. p.55

> Pathology that is seen to be associated with *social stresses*, fear, anxiety, insecurity, and (gradually) the establishment of (a state of) depression are the results of water deficiency to the point that the water requirement of brain tissue (brain cells) is affected. The brain uses electrical energy that is generated by the presence of water. With dehydration, the level of energy generation in the brain is decreased. Many functions of the brain that depend upon this (water-generated) energy become inefficient. We recognize (the symptoms associated with) this inadequacy of function and call it *depression*. p.57

> Dehydration is the number one stressor of the human body. Chronic cellular dehydration painfully and prematurely kills. Its initial outward manifestations have until now been labeled as diseases of unknown origin. p.69

Section 1 - Getting Ready

I read the entire book on the flight home. I couldn't put it down. First thing on Monday morning I called the publisher listed in the front of the book, hoping to make a telephone appointment with Dr. Batmanghelidj (known to his legion of devoted fans as Dr. B). To my utter surprise and delight, I was told to hold the line and within a minute or so I was talking to Dr. B. himself. He was very generous with his time. He was very patient with my questions and my skepticism. He kept repeating himself over and over again. "Just follow the watercure recipe and you will be fine." Two hours went by. I finally agreed to follow the guidelines of his watercure recipe. I told him I would stay in touch and let him know if anything positive happened. I hung up the phone and started the watercure.

Prior to that moment, I never drank more than one or two glasses of water a day. And I loved water! Since the mid 1970s I had always made sure I was drinking natural spring water or purified water from a home water filter. I was always careful about my drinking and cooking water *quality*. I just never paid attention to my drinking water *quantity*. I had been taught that it didn't matter. And I believed it. I had been taught that more than enough water was in my cooked whole grains and steamed vegetables and fresh fruits. I was taught to "eat when you're hungry and drink when you're thirsty." And so I did. For about 25 years I drank one or two glasses of water a day. Dr. B was claiming that at my size and body weight (six foot tall and 200 pounds), I needed about six times that amount on a daily basis. There was no way I could consume that much water. There simply wouldn't be any room for anything else! Or so I thought.

I had to accept something very important and very real. No matter what I thought about drinking that much water, the simple fact of the matter was I had never consumed that much water before and I had been experiencing bouts of depression and anxiety off and on for the past 25 years! I had run out of ideas myself and nobody else in my life was coming up with any new ideas. I had absolutely nothing to lose and potentially everything in the world to gain. I tried it. Fourteen days later my depression lifted and has not returned since. Not once. I have not had one moment of acute anxiety, and not one panic attack since either. Oh, yeah. And no more kidney stones!

Imagine that.

The habit of proper daily hydration according to the guidelines set up by Dr. B in his (soon to be more) famous watercure recipe was the last piece of a puzzle that I had been searching for, for a very long time. In the seventeen years that have passed since my initial discovery

Section 1 - Getting Ready

of the watercure, I have not missed one day of following that recipe. I encourage you to do the same thing. I have tried to the best of my ability to share the watercure with everyone I know. There is nothing that I have discovered in over 40 years of searching for common sense health solutions more important than the watercure. The watercure may turn out to be the single most important health discovery of all time.

Imagine that. (The watercure recipe is found on page 120.)

Thank you for reading my story. I hope you enjoyed it. I hope you learned something. Please read the other stories I have included here in the final pages of Section One. I know that you are eager to get to the other parts of the *Intestinal Regeneration Program* found in Section Two. I am eager for you to get there too. Simply keep in mind that each one of the next six stories was carefully chosen with you in mind. Remember that each story is a true story, a case history report from a recent client of mine who is following the same program I am describing to you in this book. I believe there is a powerful seed of truth for you in each of the next six stories. A truth that could set you free from the pain and suffering of your current digestive system problems.

Russell Mariani

South Hadley, Massachusetts

March, 2006.

Even in our sleep, pain, which we cannot forget,
falls drop by drop upon the heart, until in despair,
against our own will, comes wisdom.
Aeschylus.

Note from RM: In July, 2014 I am happy to report that almost everything in my own diet and lifestyle remains the same and that means that the basic components of my Intestinal Regeneration Program remain the same with only slight modifications here and there and these changes are reflected in the updated and revised 2014 version of Healing Digestive Illness which you are reading right now.

Grant's Story: Ulcerative Colitis

In the summer of 2004, it had been 31 years since my own experience with ulcerative colitis. One day I received a phone call from a young man named Grant. He was 22 years old and had been suffering from ulcerative colitis for almost four years. He was at his wit's end and on the verge of a nervous breakdown. His life had become totally unbearable to him. As he described his symptoms and condition to me over the phone, so much of what he had been suffering from reminded me of my own experiences so many years ago. As he started to get better soon after following my suggestions, I knew it was time for me to write this book. I started writing this book in September of 2004. RM

Here is Grant's story in his own words:
At the start of my sophomore year of college I began to notice blood on my toilet tissue. At the time I felt healthy and decided to continue on with my normal business, which meant ignoring the situation. I took this approach for about three months until I began to notice that my bleeding was progressively getting worse. I began to get really worried for I knew that the sight of blood in a bowel movement was not a normal part of the process. I didn't know what it meant, but I knew it wasn't good. I discussed the situation with my parents and they immediately set up an appointment with a gastroenterologist (GI doctor) to have the situation checked out. The GI doctor performed a sigmoidoscopy and told me that I had a *mild case* of proctitis and that it wasn't anything serious and I didn't need to worry about it.

Out of curiosity I began to question the doctor as to the cause of the proctitis and whether this condition could lead to anything more serious down the road. The doctor told me that they didn't know what caused the bleeding and the best thing for me to do was to take anti-inflammatory suppositories and just forget about it. Relieved that my situation wasn't more serious, I continued on with my life as a regular college student.

Gradually, over the course of the next several months I began to see more and more blood in my stool and I started to get terrible cramps in my gut. I went back to my GI doctor and expressed concern that my proctitis seemed to be getting worse. He assured me that *the cause was unknown* and that the only thing that he could do was to prescribe more suppositories. *I felt an overwhelming innate sense* that my proctitis had a simple solution and that the doctor was leading me down the wrong road. As I began my junior year in college the blood in my stool was increasing, my gut began cramping severely, and I was battling constant fatigue.

I could no longer participate in the active lifestyle that I was accustomed to and became extremely discouraged. My parents made an appointment with our family physician to see if he could offer any suggestions about relieving my discomfort and fatigue. I explained to the physician how bad my situation had become over the past year and how it was ruining my life. He told me to bend over and he gave me the old rubber glove treatment. He told me that proctitis was a general term and that I probably just had a hemorrhoid. Like the previous doctor he told me that I should take an anti-inflammatory suppository and to just forget about it.

I explained to him that I had been taking suppositories for many months and that they were not working. He got defensive. He told me that *he* was the medical professional and that *I* should just listen to his advice and not self-diagnose.

Discouraged after my visits to the first two doctors, I went to another GI doctor who performed another sigmoidoscopy and gave me a new diagnosis: *Ulcerative Colitis*. He told me that this was an *auto-immune disease* and that there was no cure, an answer that I really didn't want to hear, considering the fact that I was 21 years old and didn't want to live with this painful and distressing ailment for the rest of my life. This doctor then prescribed an enema product called *Rowasa*, and the drug *Coloxyl*, in an attempt to control my symptoms and alleviate some of the pain. I took these drugs for three months and saw no improvement in my condition.

As a result of taking these newest drugs, the only thing I noticed was that the pain and bloating in my stomach seemed to have become worse. *I asked whether diet was a possible cause and the doctor said that diet had nothing to do with it.* He told me that I should eat a well-balanced standard American diet, but he gave no direction or guidance as to what a well-balanced standard American diet was. As I left his office I felt as if the medical community was really letting me down. They were not being helpful at all, but rather than apologizing for not being able (or willing!) to answer my questions or reduce my pain and discomfort, they made me feel that it was all my fault, and worst of all, that my symptoms might just be the result of "my thinking or emotions" that somehow, it was all in my head. What, as if I were making all this up to get their attention? Right.

I finally decided to take matters into my own hands and started researching ulcerative colitis on my own. I decided to give certain diets a try to see if I could get my *incurable* condition to improve. I experimented with paleo-diets, low-carb diets, vegetarian diets, and even a strict raw food diet. Nothing worked. I kept getting worse.

Out of deep concern for my health, my parents forced me to go back to the GI doctor who always said the same thing: "We don't know the cause" and that "you should just eat a well-balanced standard American diet." This time, however, he added something new. *He said that I shouldn't worry because if things continued to get worse he could give me immune suppressing steroid drugs and if necessary he could just remove the problematic sections of my colon.* This did not seem like a proper solution to me at all.

I struggled my way through my last semester of college and ended up graduating, but I was so debilitated by that point in my life that I could barely make it to my final exams. I actually missed my graduation ceremony because I couldn't leave the toilet for more than thirty minutes at a time. My parents were getting increasingly scared as they saw my once big, strong, athletic body wither away, and my emotional health along with it. Hey, I was scared too! I went to chiropractors, acupuncturists, herbalists, massage therapists, yoga professionals, anyone I could think of that might help my condition improve at all.

The proctitis that I was told was nothing to worry about had evolved into a monster that was destroying my life and leaving me with an overwhelming sense of hopelessness. I finally reached a point where I couldn't leave my apartment and would spend the majority of the day on the toilet and then curled up in my bed in pain. Out of desperation, my mother contacted a family friend and neighbor, Scott Ohlgren, who is a natural health educator and writer. He recommended that I call Russell Mariani.

I found out that Russell had healed himself from ulcerative colitis (back in 1973) and that he had a great success record helping people with all kinds of intestinal problems. After the first ten minutes of my first conversation with Russell my spirits were lifted and I knew that this guy knew what he was talking about. Instead of giving me more hyperbole about how ulcerative colitis was an *autoimmune disease with no cure*, he started to explain to me how my digestive system is supposed to function. He then explained that one of the causes of ulcerative colitis is the depletion of the mucus lining of my colon from years of dry, hard and difficult-to-pass stools. He talked about dehydration and probiotics. He talked about whole foods, acid and alkaline, and the kind of dietary fiber that would begin to gently restore the lining of my colon. It all made sense to me.

Russell had me change my eating habits and almost instantaneously my cramping and discomfort were gone and my bowels began to function properly for the first time in years. I felt relief in a matter of days. After just three weeks of working with Russell, I was confident that my years of suffering were a thing of the past. At this writing it has been six months and I am completely pain-free and symptom-free. My "incurable ulcerative colitis" is nowhere to be found. I'm baffled and angry that I had to endure years of pain and misery because the medical profession apparently didn't know what they were talking about. They led me down the wrong road while destroying my hopes of ever healing my condition. What is up with that?

I feel extremely fortunate that circumstances led me to Russell. Without the nutritional guidance and weekly coaching and support from him, I would be living a nightmare of pain, misery, and hopelessness. I know that there are thousands of other individuals in the same situation that I was in and I can only pray that they are eventually presented with a similar opportunity to get well.

The moral of my story? Don't ever let anyone make you believe that there is no cure and that you have to live with the pain and discomfort of ulcerative colitis for the rest of your life (or any other digestive system problem). The key to wellness is proper nutrition and learning about and then practicing the fundamentals of natural health!

Grant
December, 2004
(last name withheld by request)

Section 1 - Getting Ready

Brittany's Story: Extreme Constipation

I had been dealing with constipation for about a year. I was constantly uncomfortable and irritable. I would go through phases where I didn't eat for three or four days, with the thought that if it doesn't go in, it doesn't have to come out. But when I wouldn't eat I had no strength and I couldn't concentrate. Stool softeners and laxatives worked in the beginning but eventually had no effect on me. I had a *colonoscopy* and they couldn't find anything wrong. I soon relied on enemas to solve the problem. I never had a bowel movement without the help of an enema. Soon enemas stopped helping. I went to the gastrointestinal doctor. He had me swallow a pill with tiny rings in it and every three days I'd go to the hospital for x-rays. They wanted to see if the rings moved through my system. A week and a half later they told me the rings had not moved. At this point I had not had a bowel movement in over four weeks. *The doctor told me that my colon was not working AT ALL.* It was totally stopped. He told me that if I wanted to get it moving again, I'd have to have two feet of my colon removed with surgery.

I am 19 years old. I had been uncomfortable for so long that I agreed with the idea. If it would work, then I would do it. I had tried so many things. I did so many kinds of herbs, laxatives, fiber, stool softeners, enemas, mineral oil, and much more. That night we came home from the surgeon's office, my Mom didn't go to bed. She was still on the internet when I woke up the next morning. She found Russell's website. She noticed that he had been successful with people who suffered with constipation problems. She said she wanted me to try to get help from him before I talked again to the surgeon. I was frustrated. I had tried so

Section 1 - Getting Ready

many things with no success and now she was pushing another one on me. Russell promised my Mom that his program would work. I wasn't sure at all.

To be honest, I was very doubtful. But Russell sounded so relaxed and confident that I decided to try his program. I started taking the intestinal herb capsules and doing the water treatment. About a week later I had my first bowel movement. I can't tell you how excited I was! Excited about being able to poop. I'd have bowel movements about every other day. Eventually I started having them about twice a day. It's been over a month now and I just can't believe how normal everything is, better than it's ever been. I'm so glad my Mom found Russell. If she didn't I'd now have part of my colon removed and who knows if that would have helped or not.

Brittany

April 5, 2004

(last name withheld by request)

Here's a letter I got from Brittany's Mom on May 20, 2004.

Dear Russell,

I just wanted to express my appreciation for your help. As you well know, three months ago, we were at a total loss as to what to do about Britt's extreme constipation. The one thing I did know was that removing part of her bowel was not the answer we were looking for! I know that you have talked to her on the phone and she tells you she is feeling better but what she probably hasn't told you is how much better she looks. Her skin tones look much healthier and she has that sparkle back in her eyes. Although she's not gained any weight (she didn't need to) her body doesn't look gaunt and unhealthy anymore. (At the time of her wedding, I was very concerned about her weight. People asked me daily why she was getting so thin.) I know she wasn't eating right at all, because her theory was, if something goes in, something must come out, and as you know, that wasn't happening at all. I'm truly grateful that I found your name after doing a google search on the internet. I honestly believe that things happen for a reason and in finding you, we found the answer to our prayers.

Many thanks again and God Bless!

Sincerely,

Brittany's Mom

(name withheld by request)

Section 1 - Getting Ready

Mike's Story: Crohn's Disease

I *was* a Crohn's sufferer; with most of the *usual suspects* as symptoms: severe abdominal pain, diarrhea, weight loss, no energy, no appetite, and an overall feeling of impending doom: *like I'd never be well again*! I started my treatment journey in the standard medical way since I knew no other way at the time; prednisone, sulfur drugs, immuran. This regimen covered up my symptoms about four days a week, but the other three days I was sick. (Same old symptoms!) This was all happening in the early part of 1986. I had my first surgery about a year later to remove 10 cm (about three inches) of my small intestine. The surgery gave me roughly two symptom-free years. But drugs and surgery did not address the underlying causes of my condition. In time, my symptoms returned and I was back on the drug-wagon again. I experienced peaks, valleys, and all the adverse side effects; pain, nausea, a swollen-puffy-blown-up-looking face, the shakes, mood swings, animal-like hunger one day, no appetite the next. The list of symptoms was endless.

Another surgery followed after my small intestine perforated in 1995, and the doctors had to remove another 10 cm of small intestine. This time, I was marginally better for only about three months, then the roof caved in again. My negative symptoms reached a new low that I didn't think was possible. I went to the experts at Mt. Sinai (a hospital in New York City) and another regime of drugs was prescribed: Prednisone, Pentasa, 6mp, Cipro. I wept at night believing I would never be well again. My wife, though supportive, felt as if our lives were being taken from us.

Section 1 - Getting Ready

On my knees one night, praying, I gave it all to God. I gave up. I surrendered. I told Him that I couldn't go on and asked for His mercy. I asked Him to take this burden of my illness away from me. That was the catalyst that gave me new vigor and energy to find another way... His way. In my surrendering to God, something wonderful happened. Something changed. I felt hopeful again. I had the energy to search for answers and to take personal responsibility for my own healing. I was beginning to understand the difference between true healing and covering up my symptoms with drugs and surgery.

I started fiddling with my diet, and paying more attention to my lifestyle. I didn't really know what I was doing. I simply knew that I had to make changes. Staying the same and doing the same old, same old, was just making me sicker and sicker. I knew that standard medical treatment was not making me well, it was making me sicker. I was now open to finding a better way to health; I just didn't know what that way was going to be.

Then, at a health seminar in April 2003, I met Russell. I sat and listened to his personal story about healing from colitis. (He said he was originally misdiagnosed with colon cancer.) This motivated me and gave me even more energy and drive to be rid of my disease. After the seminar I contacted him via telephone and starting following his suggestions right away. I made changes in my diet and lifestyle and added some nutritional supplements to my daily routine. He taught me what was really happening in my gut and that bowel disorders were diseases of the fork.

The dietary changes I made were simple ones: whole foods instead of processed foods, proper daily hydration, probiotic supplements, chewing my food. My friends and family were concerned with all my new and *weird* habits, but I could tell it was all working for me within a matter of days. I agreed to give this program my full commitment for 90 days. Wonderful things began to happen. The fire in my bowels became quiet and cool. I started having normal and regular bowel movements for the first time in years. When my disease was active, it was normal for me to have to visit the bathroom 10 to 15 times a day. My energy levels increased and I was beginning to feel empowered and that I could lick this ugly thing for good. I pushed on, and felt stronger and stronger. I began to *take myself* off the drugs one by one; first the Prednisone, very slowly, then the others. My mental clarity and increasing sense of personal freedom were indescribable. I was able to concentrate on my family and work without having to think about Crohn's disease for the first time ever. Ah, this was how normal people lived!

After a few months, I was feeling so good that I got a little cocky. I made the mistake in thinking that since my symptoms were gone, that I could go back to all the junk food I had missed. My mistake was in not truly understanding that it was all that junk food and other habits that had caused my Crohn's disease in the first place. *It was a hard lesson to learn, but one of the most important in my life so far.* Now I know what I need to do to keep my digestive system functioning properly. I want to do the things that nourish me best, and allow my body to continue to get stronger and stronger and stronger. Do I miss certain foods? Sure I do, but not half as much as I miss all those nasty symptoms associated with Crohn's. I do not miss all the adverse side effects of all those drugs either. *I do not miss Zombie Mike at all*! Besides, as I get healthier and stronger, I'm certain my diet will become more and more varied not less and less so. I am still in the earliest stages of recovery and healing. I am learning that health is about freedom not restriction. I am feeling more and more comfortable in my own body and more and more confident that I am on the right path. I feel great!

I recently went to my family doctor for a full physical exam. He asked me what drugs I was taking and I told him none. When he had last seen me I was in pretty bad shape, taking lots of different drugs. He drew some blood that day. I told him that once I changed my diet and lifestyle and took the supplements, wonderful things began to happen and that I was feeling terrific for the first time in a very long time. He said: "*I don't believe in that stuff. It was your surgery nine years ago that made you well.*" I then asked him to explain how I was able to get off all the drugs and why I was feeling so normal. He had no explanation. I got my blood test results a week later which revealed a sedimentation rate of 4, (the degree of inflammation in my body) and a complete blood test of *totally normal readings*. Once again, the doctor had no explanation. But I knew exactly what I had done to allow my body to heal itself. To me, it's as plain and as logical as adding two plus two and getting four. Why my doctor doesn't see this is a strange mystery to me.

Shortly thereafter, I had a series of x-rays taken to see what was going on inside my small intestine. In my previous series taken two years earlier, it was revealed that I had a three inch section of Crohn's disease on the ileum side of the hookup between my small and large intestine (near the ileo-cecal valve). I also had some Crohn's narrowing in the mid-section of my gut. Well, the new results were pretty amazing to say the least. The narrowing in the mid-section of my gut was *no longer detectable!* The only narrowing they could find was a 3 cm area (1 inch) of Crohn's near the ileo-cecal valve. And this small area was no longer inflamed or active. It appears to me that my intestines are physically regenerating themselves: with my cooperation of course!

Today I am in control. I am properly educated about my disease and feeling personally empowered about how to be well and stay well. I thank God and I praise God every single day for the grace I have received to more fully understand that in this life and on this earth, my body is the temple for His holy spirit. By eating healthier foods and practicing sensible, enjoyable lifestyle habits, I am experiencing the benefits of physical regeneration, spiritual renewal and personal healing. How sweet it is!

Mike Roscigno, Long Valley, New Jersey, March 24, 2004

An important update to Mike's Story:
Fast forward: Summer 2004

I had been hearing of the fantastic results that others were getting with a new drug on the market called Remicade. People were astounded at the increases in lifestyle, energy boost, weight gain, you name it. I fell for it, hook, line and sinker. Why the heck not, it almost sounded like you could forget your disease and be "normal again." Why was I tempted? Because I missed my old food habits! Can you believe it? Old habits die hard and if truth be told I did not fully understand the relationship between food and healing. Even after everything I had been through. So, I dove right in. Two infusions later, I had the surge in weight gain, positive feelings of no more Crohn's, then the floor gave way.

The 16 pounds I gained faded gradually over a few months. The symptoms returned, and that one inch area near my ileo-cecal value acted like a brick wall. Not much food/waste was getting through. What I went on to learn is that in areas of previous narrowing, the Remicade will produce some healing AND additional scar tissue in areas of active disease. In my case, my one inch area that I was able to manage previously was now mostly scar tissue and an area of big concern since no natural, medical or food regimen could open it up. So here we go again, the only way to open the gates again was another surgery. This one was not as bad as the others because the Doc's were able to perform it laparoscopically and I was in and out of the "big house" in 4 days.

A new record according to the esteemed AMA establishment. Wow! Problem was I gave up another 5 inches of my intestine. See, those of you that have been down this road know that the surgeons usually take an inch on either side of the diseased area and also in my case they had to take 2 inches of my large intestine for the new "hookup." Don't let the big boys fool you. They say you've got a zillion feet of intestine and you can still function normally without a very big chunk of it. Well, maybe. Fact remains that whatever they take out is no longer available to you to absorb needed nutrients for proper, normal living. At risk now are hemoglobin counts, B12 levels, anemia, total proteins, iron….you name it. So, DON'T do it unless it is life threatening. There are other, better ways and I've already documented some previously in this story.

So, here I was back at square one. Or so it seemed. Now it was the summer of 2005. Frustrated and angry, my bowel shorter and not feeling so great after the surgery. It was crunch time again. Time to dig in your heels, look right down the barrel of the disease and be one track minded to be a winner again and to beat this thing.

I was DETERMINED TO NEVER be in a position like this ever again. I was damn sick of co-payments, lab tests, frequent trips to the pharmacy, seeing Doctors. I have literally grown to despise the medical establishment. Not the people. They are all sensitive, respectful, mostly knowledgeable people but they don't know jack about how best to treat this disease.

I started again by creating an environment for healing in my bowel with a number of natural herbal formulas that worked. I then began to eat like people who don't have a history of bowel disease in their country, like the Japanese. Organic brown rice porridge and miso soup for breakfast along with a Superfood regimen of a powerful green drink mixed with carrot juice I squeeze myself or some blue green algae supplements along with probiotics. Boom. Here goes the energy and confidence up, up, up and away!

Virtually eliminating ALL animal food and not putting any undue strain on the bowels by eating any large meals. I started practicing all the fundamentals again that I had learned from Russell and his Intestinal Regeneration Program.

And this is the missing link for me; physical training that never stops. Exercise! Constant and never ending focus on training the body, keep it moving and be determined to bring out the best that God intended for you. Hire a trainer, get a family member to whack you over the head every other day. Whatever it takes, do it! It will change your life. Believe me, when you look in the mirror at night after getting out of the shower and see the changes, it energizes you like never before.

So, here I am, in control, feeling empowered again and building a new body. The feeling is exhilarating. Getting that attitude makes you look at life in a whole new way. So go on, get it done now. You'll never look back!

Mike Roscigno
July, 2006

Maxine's Story: Acute Diverticulitis

As a woman's health-care nurse-practitioner, I never realized the severity of my acute diverticulitis in August, 2003. Due to a high tolerance for pain I thought I had a simple urinary tract infection. After that test proved negative, I ended up having a CTScan. In fact I ended up having three CTScans, at a cost of over $5,000 to assess the source of my pain. (Due to my high tolerance to pain, the only way to assess my condition/progress was by CTScan.) The doctors found that I had acute diverticulitis with fistulas extending from the sigmoid colon to the rectum. I was advised to go from the CTScan department via my surgeon to the operating room, at which time I was supposed to have six inches of my intestines removed (from the descending colon) and to get a colostomy bag. Instead of surgery, I found Russell, through a mutual friend, Joanne Dinnie (head GI nurse at Baystate Medical Center, in Springfield, Massachusetts). *Russell, in my opinion, is a bowel health genius.* After just five weeks following his program I felt almost fully recovered. A colonoscopy done in December 2003 showed no inflammation at all. I have no doubt that as long as I continue to do the things I have learned from Russell, my intestinal condition will continue to improve and regenerate. It is now July 2004, and I continue to consult with him on a regular basis. I have no pain and I am symptom-free.

Maxine Costa, RN MSN/BSN/APRN

Note: It is now March, 2006 and I continue to speak with Maxine on a regular basis. She continues to be pain-free and symptom free. She is doing just great! Now our conversations focus primarily on the referrals she sends me from the two women's health care centers where she works. RM

Section 1 - Getting Ready

🌰 Bob's Story: IBS, Acid Reflux, and Much More!

I had been experiencing a number of health problems that seemed to be slowly getting worse over a period of several years. The most significant problems were in three categories: 1. Digestive Problems. I had heartburn, gas, indigestion, stomach cramps and occasional diarrhea. 2. Skeletal-Muscular Problems. I had constant muscle soreness and stiffness. I developed arthritis in my back, neck and hip. 3. Immune System Problems. I would have frequent sinus infections, sore throats, coughing spells and body aches. I saw my physician on a regular basis for all these problems, but aside from confirming a diagnosis of arthritis, any blood tests taken always came back negative. I am only 48 years old and have enjoyed playing basketball for many years, but that has become increasingly difficult and less and less enjoyable to do. As I looked ahead, I just couldn't imagine my life with all these health problems. It just seemed like things would continue to get worse and worse unless I came up with a different strategy.

In addition to all of the above, I had been experiencing frequent headaches, fatigue and shaking of my hands. Now that I have had some time to reflect upon all this, I realize that my digestive problems go back to my teenage years. I was always a compulsive eater, and a regular over-eater, day after day after day. I remember feeling hungry most of the time, but even when I wasn't hungry, I still felt driven to eat compulsively.

When my hands started shaking and I experienced soreness in my kidney area and behind my neck, I made a decision to figure out what were the causes of all these problems. Conventional medicine was able to identify the onset of arthritis, and took note of my general body stiffness, but was unable to identify the cause of anything or make any connections between and among any of my symptoms. This made less and less sense to me.

I went to my chiropractor to get his opinion about my physical problems related to the body stiffness, muscle soreness, and fatigue. He asked whether I had any digestive system problems. I told him that I did. At that point he recommended that I see Russell. The rest as they say is history. I started working with Russell in March 2004.

All of the digestive problems I had were effectively eliminated within a very short period of time. I have not had a full-blown sinus infection or other significant illness since we started working together. My muscle soreness has been reduced. I continue to work to reduce my stiffness and arthritis. I have made a lot of progress in this area and I am eager to make even greater progress in the months ahead.

What I have learned by working with Russell is that there are certain complementary habits that when practiced, allow the body's own natural processes to maintain optimal health. There are also insulting habits that when indulged on a regular basis will interfere with the body's own natural processes and invite many problems and difficulties. I have incorporated the following complementary habits into my current diet and lifestyle:

1. The Watercure.
2. Effective Supplements before every meal.
3. I eat more consciously. I chew more thoroughly.
4. I am gradually reducing the frequency of certain insulting habits and/or eliminating them altogether.
5. I am eating more whole foods and less processed foods.
6. I have learned the importance of seasonal cleansing of certain organs: liver, colon, kidneys.
7. I have learned the importance of something I have come to name, *reflective practice.* By reflective practice I mean being more aware of how my own body responds to the things I do, and to make a greater effort to be less mechanical and reactive and more conscious and responsive in what I do.

I have found that the concepts of complementary and insulting habits and reflective practice are general principles that I have tried to apply to other aspects of my life. Whether it be physical exercise, work, eating, or relationships, it seems to me that there are complementary habits and insulting habits that are related to all these activities; in fact to all possible activities.

We need to acquire knowledge so that we can begin to make the distinctions between complementary and insulting habits. We then need to acquire the knowledge about the most effective ways to practice the complementary habits. Lastly, we need to understand what prevents us from acting upon such knowledge because this inaction is at the root cause of much suffering in our world today. *Reflective practice is necessary in order to adapt to the particular needs of your own unique situation.* Just as no two bodies are exactly alike, no two situations are exactly alike, and so we must take responsibility for adapting the wisdom that is passed along to us.

I can just imagine what my life would be like today, if I had not placed that first phone call to Russell. All those years I suffered! I hope that many others will find out about the things that I have recently discovered to turn my own health around. I hope my story helps. I hope my story will encourage others to take action and find out the difference between complementary and insulting habits. I hope others will take the actions that are necessary to discover the things that nourish them best.

Bob Dufresne, November, 2004

Robert J. Dufresne, PhD.

CEO, Pioneer Valley Educational Press

Amherst, Massachusetts 01003

Please check out Bob's very helpful essay about *Reflective Practice* which appears on page 201. Bob is a devoted husband and father of two sons. He is a trained physicist and has worked in the field of education as a researcher and in curriculum development for over 25 years.

Section 1 - Getting Ready

Jessica's Story:
Extreme Gas and Bloating

I am a thirty-something year old accountant and don't think I write very well but I wanted to share my story anyway.

I was diagnosed a few years ago with IBS by a gastroenterologist. I took Zelnorm and Miralax for over a year and they didn't help at all. My condition was that I was severely constipated and extremely gassy. I had to take prescription laxatives to get any movement from my bowels, but nothing I ever did was really very effective and it felt like I was just playing games, and my intestines were always losing. I got extremely bloated with intestinal gas every single day. It would start right after breakfast. By the time I would get to work I would be so swollen and uncomfortable that I would have to unbutton my pants. After lunch it only got worse. I felt like my stomach was swollen as big as a basketball. I had to run to the restroom every twenty minutes just to sit down on the toilet and let out the gas. I was so uncomfortable all the time. I couldn't wait to get out of work and get home and put on my sweatpants. This was my daily routine for years.

I started working with Russell Mariani in September 2004, after much encouragement from my gynecologist, Maxine Costa. She knew about my problems for years, and she had worked with Russell directly on some digestive problems of her own. After much procrastination, I finally called. I was so miserable and uncomfortable, and nothing else was working. I had to try something different.

Russell walked me through my first official colon cleanse. Actually he talked me through it over the phone. He taught me about proper daily hydration and introduced me to probiotics and what to eat for breakfast

Section 1 - Getting Ready

and what not to eat for breakfast. He taught me the importance of eating more slowly and deliberately and really chewing my food.

Within a few short weeks all the gas and bloating were gone. No more basketball size belly. No more running to the restroom at work every twenty minutes. No more unbearable pain and discomfort. I started having regular daily bowel movements for the first time in years. I know exactly what to do to maintain my great intestinal condition and how to prevent problems from happening again in the future. I can't tell you how excited I am to have finally solved these problems. And I know at least one other person who is excited too… my fiance. I will be getting married in the spring of 2005!

Russell's *Intestinal Regeneration Program* works. It's simple. I am so glad that I don't have to spend the rest of my life in such pain and discomfort. It feels so good to have a normal, quiet, happy belly!

Jessica (last name withheld by request.)
December, 2004

For recent updates on all these people and their stories and to read more stories from other people go to: www.healingdigestiveillness.com

Section 1 - Getting Ready

Your Story:
Five Vital Question Areas

Now it's time to focus on *your story*. Your story is composed of the answers to five vital question areas (see below). Some of these answers you know already. Some of these answers you will learn by reading this book. All of these answers will be very clear to you, in a few months time, after you have been practicing the complementary dietary and lifestyle habits presented in this book. Please take a few minutes now to put down the answers to as many of these questions as you feel comfortable answering today. *I suggest that you answer all of them, one at a time.* And remember, this is not a test. There are no wrong answers. Just your answers. I would suggest that you print this page out (or make a photo-copy) and write down your answers and save them. You will want to compare them to your answers a few weeks or a few months down the road, when you are feeling 100% better than you are feeling today. You may be surprised at how much you already knew. You may be surprised at how much new stuff that you have learned. Perhaps you will not be surprised at all. Nevertheless, this is an important exercise to do, and this will be the last thing to do, before learning about the specifics of your *Intestinal Regeneration Program* in the next section.

The Five Vital Question Areas:

As they relate to your overall health and well-being and the many factors in your diet and lifestyle. Use as much space as you need to answer each of the following questions completely.

Section 1 - Getting Ready

1. Where are you right now? What is your current condition? Have you been given a medical diagnosis for your condition? What are your primary symptoms? What are your secondary symptoms? Do you think they are related or not? Do you have any other symptoms anywhere else in your body not already mentioned? How would you describe your current mental/emotional/psychological state? (happy, sad, curious, complacent, angry, frustrated, disappointed, etc) On a scale of 1-10 (10 being perfectly healthy, 1 being dead) how would you assess the quality of your overall health and well-being today?

2. How did you get here? How long have you been suffering these various symptoms and primary condition? When did these symptoms first begin to manifest in your life? Do you have any insights into the cause or causes of your symptoms and condition? Have you had any accident, injury, or illness in the past that may be contributing to your current symptoms and condition? Is there any relevant personal medical history? Is there any relevant family medical history? What are your best guesses as to what factors/habits/influences have caused your current condition?

3. Where do you want to go? Imagine you had Aladdin's Lamp. What three wishes would you ask for, related to your current health condition? Imagine you are perfectly healthy. Describe your new symptoms of health. What does your life look like as a result of being perfectly healthy and symptom-free? What is your deepest desire as it relates to your current state of health?

4. What are your compelling reasons to change? Where do you think you will be one year from now if you don't find the solutions to your current health challenges? Is there anyone in your life who depends on you to be healthy and energetic? How does your current condition and symptoms affect your relationships with the people you love and care about the most? What happens if you don't get better? Why must you find effective solutions to your current health challenges? Why must you get better? Answer these questions with emotion and conviction. And by the way, what is the purpose of your life? Why are you here on this earth at this time?

5. What is your Plan? What is your plan to get from where you are right now to where you want to be? Do you have a reliable map, compass, and experienced guide? As the old saying goes; "If you don't know where you're going, you'll probably end up somewhere else!" What is your plan? Can you get there from here? Are you sure?

Section Two
GETTING STARTED

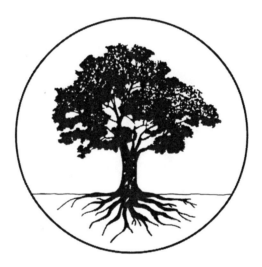

Food is the soil from which the tree of our own life is grown.

Section 2 - Getting Started

🌰 *Introduction to Section Two*

It's time to change gears. All the preliminaries are over. I am going to assume that you have turned to this section because you are serious about correcting your digestive system problems and you are ready to activate my suggestions and integrate the steps of this program with 100% commitment. If you are not ready to give it your 100% attention and commitment, then please, don't bother. Go do something else. Don't waste your precious time, money, energy and other valuable resources. I am not interested in creating more problems for you. I am not interested in creating yet another health "program" you tried, that you say didn't work. *I am interested in helping you to permanently solve your digestive system problems.* I can assure you that this program works, but you have to work the program correctly. Working the program correctly means working it with understanding. Understanding requires reading, studying, processing, acceptance.

Acceptance of what? The acceptance of the basic fact that your body knows exactly how to heal itself as long as you are cooperating consciously and consistently as described in Section One. This program should make sense to you based upon what you have already read so far. With understanding and acceptance it will be much easier to cooperate, be consistent and stay committed. These are the keys to producing desirable results.

If you need some more convincing before you are ready to give me 100% of your attention and commitment, I have a few suggestions for you. Go back to the beginning of the book and start reading it all over again from page 1. Read every paragraph and every page. Read it word for word. How does it make you feel? What does it make you think about? Read it with a pen and a hi-liter and a notebook. Take notes. Then, actually take the time to read your own notes. Read through the testimonials again. And then read through the testimonials, again. Do not skim. Do not scan. Do not speed-read. The testimonials are not made-up or made-over. *They are written by people just like you.* The success they achieved is directly proportional to how and why they implemented this program. They were willing to make whatever adjustments they needed to make along the way, until they got it right. These adjustments are built into the program. They are explained completely throughout the rest of this book, but you have to pay attention in order to discover when they apply to you and your situation. You have to pay attention to what is going on inside you own body in order to determine what adjustments you will need to make and when, and where, and how and why. This is just common sense.

I want you to get fantastic results from this program. I am committed to doing everything I can at my end to make sure you get fantastic results. You just have to play your part. Just follow my suggestions. Take one step at a time. Be patient. Use common sense. Pay attention. Be flexible. Be smart. Don't make the mistake of looking at my suggestions, narrowly focus on one or two of them, and, based on past experience or no experience, or someone else's experience or opinion, decide: "that does not or will not work for me." I have heard all these comments and opinions hundreds of times before. I haven't worked with anyone who hasn't tried a million other things before finding me. I haven't worked with anyone who hasn't been filled with skepticism, doubt, and fear based upon all their past experiences in seeking effective solutions for his or her digestive system problems.

I know that some of you have already tried one or two of the components of this program and you do have some direct experience that the things you have tried have not worked.

I totally understand this. I totally understand your frustration. I totally understand your skepticism, doubt, fear, anger. I simply invite you to consider something: You have not yet worked directly with me and my program. You have not yet invested the time, money resources and energy into integrating all the components of my program into your diet and into your lifestyle. This may seem like a small thing. It's not. This distinction makes all the difference in the world. Understanding this distinction is the key to your success with this program. I see it every day. Not a day goes by in my private practice where I am not clearly reminded of the absolute importance of the synergistic benefits of the whole program over any of its parts or any other combination of its parts.

One part of the program does not equal the whole program. Several parts of the program do not equal the whole program. The whole program works successfully when all of the parts are integrated fully and completely. When all the parts are integrated effectively your body activates a powerful biological principle called *synergy*. The definition of synergy is this: *The whole is much greater than the mere sum of the parts*. Consistent physical regeneration will not start happening in your body until this phenomenon of synergy gets properly activated. The best way to properly activate the principle of synergy available to you through this *Intestinal Regeneration Program* is to implement every part of this program with consistency and commitment.

The key to the effectiveness of this program is that it invites you to fully integrate all the most important health and nutrition fundamentals at the same time. Nothing is left out.

To the best of my knowledge, no program like mine exists. No one has put together these same components into one coherent and integrated whole. Lots of individuals and lots of practitioners have found one or more of these same components, but still do not experience relief and sustainable results. All I can tell you is this: each piece of this program has been painstakingly discovered, worked on and mastered to a very significant degree. Not one piece of this program is new. Each piece of this program has been tested over time. The last piece of this program was added in 1997 (the watercure). All the other pieces have been together for at least ten to twenty years before that.

The program works together as an integrated, synergistic whole. If you leave one piece out, it may not work. If you think one part of the program is more important than another part, it may not work. If you replace the products I suggest with other products, it may not work. If you understand that each part of the program is equally important, including the attitude with which you approach and participate in the program, you will do just fine.

Cultivate an attitude of gratitude. Miracles can and will unfold. Step into the peace of simple things. Come to know directly the power and magic of Commitment in your life.

The Healing Power of Commitment

There is nothing in our lives more powerful than commitment. Nothing unleashes more magic. Nothing turns more dreams into reality. Nothing levels the playing field more. Nothing makes the impossible more possible than commitment. Conversely, there is nothing sadder and more disappointing than people who have not yet experienced the power of commitment to heal their own conditions and transform their own lives.

I would never ask anyone, especially someone who is not feeling 100% healthy, to throw caution to the wind, and dive into my program, or anyone else's program with blind faith. I would never ask anyone to make a commitment to my program without first very carefully examining it and thinking about it. I want you to be fully aware of the importance of all your prior experiences. I want you to weigh all your current options. I want you to make a firm decision about what you are going to do *next* in your life as it relates to your current digestive system problems. I want you to make a commitment to my program, *if and only if*, it makes sense to you. I want you to make an informed decision. I want you to make an informed commitment.

I want you to read the following poem. In fact, I want you to print it out, put it on your desk or wall or bathroom mirror and over the next seven days, I want you to memorize this poem. No kidding. Consider this your first homework assignment. There will be many more *homework assignments* in the days ahead, but none more important than this one. Remember, each part of this program is equally important. Here's the poem. Please forgive the gender-biased language. The poem was written in the 1950s.

Commitment

Until one is committed there is hesitancy,
the chance to draw back, always ineffectiveness.
Concerning all acts of initiative (and creation),
there is one elementary truth, the ignorance of which
kills countless ideas and splendid plans:
that the moment one definitely commits oneself,
then Providence moves too.
All sorts of thing occur to help one
that would never otherwise have occurred.
A whole stream of events issues from the decision,
raising in one's favor all manner of unforeseen
incidents and meetings and material assistance,
which no man could have dreamt would have come his way.
I have learned a deep respect
for one of Goethe's couplets:

Whatever you can do, or dream you can, begin it.
Boldness has genius, power, and magic in it.

W.H. Murray
(The Scottish Himalayan Expedition, 1951)

The Key Problem Areas
(A Quick Review)

The problems we are seeking to correct are problems that are happening as a result of a malfunctioning digestive system. The major parts of this system include: the mouth, the throat, the esophagus, the stomach, the duodenum, the ileum, the cecum, the sigmoid colon, the rectum and the anus. The *Intestinal Regeneration Program* will address problems in all of these areas.

The named conditions or disorders or diseases associated with problems in these areas go by many different names: indigestion, acid reflux, gastroesophageal reflux disease, stomach ulcer, hernia, duodenal ulcer, Crohn's Disease, colitis, ulcerative colitis, diverticulitis, diverticulosis, proctitis, hemmorhoids, colon cancer, gastritis, Irritable Bowel Syndrome, Irritable Bowel Disorder, Inflammatory Bowel Disease, colonic inertia, constipation, candidiasis, yeast infections. The *Intestinal Regeneration Program* will address all these named conditions of the digestive system, and any other named condition of the digestive system I might have missed and you might have.

The primary symptoms associated with these named conditions include: abdominal pain, asthma, chronic joint pain, chronic muscle pain, chronic headaches, migraines, insomnia, dizziness, tinnitus (or ringing in the ears), constant coughing, sore throat, hoarseness, swelling and/or pain in the throat, gagging, frequently clearing the throat, sores on gums, lips, and tongue, mental confusion, fuzzy thinking, poor memory, anger, irritability, binge eating or drinking, poor comprehension, poor concentration, food cravings, difficulty learning, intestinal gas and bloating, indigestion, nausea, vomiting, stomach pain, cramping, heartburn, mood swings, nervousness, poor exercise

Dis-eases of the Digestive System

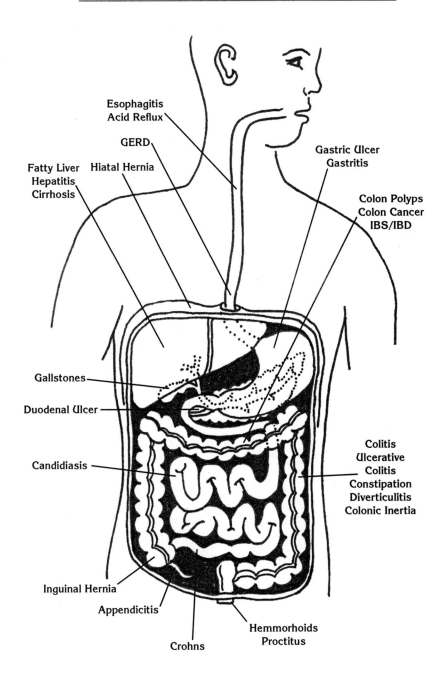

tolerance, poor immunity, recurrent vaginal infections, skin rashes, diarrhea, bed-wetting, recurrent bladder infections, fevers of unknown origin, shortness of breath, constipation, aggressive behavior, acute anxiety, easily fatigued, general malaise, chronic fatigue, depression, runny or stuffy nose, postnasal drip, buzzing in the ears, blurred vision, sinus problems, watery and itchy eyes, eye floaters, ear infections, hearing loss, sneezing attacks, hay fever, excessive mucous formation, dark circles under the eyes, swollen, red, or sticky eyelids, irregular heartbeat (palpitations, arrhythmia), rapid heartbeat, chest pain and congestion, bronchitis, shortness of breath, difficulty breathing, hives, skin rashes, psoriasis, eczema, dry skin, excessive sweating, acne, hair loss, irritation around the eyes, joint weakness, generalized weakness everywhere in the body, muscle aches and pains, arthritis, swelling, stiffness, apathy, hyperactivity, restlessness, overweight, underweight, fluid retention, genital itch, incontinence, urgent-frequent urination.

The *Intestinal Regeneration Program* will address, reduce, and eventually resolve all the uncomfortable symptoms listed above (and any others I might have missed) as long as it is applied with understanding, consistency, patience, and commitment.

🌰 Three Types of Bowel Movement Problems

There are three dominant types of bowel movements you are experiencing right now or in the most recent past. It is very important for you to recognize and then identify your condition with one of these types of bowel movements described below:

Type 1 The slow, sluggish, dry, hard, balled-up, constipated bowel movement (bm). This type will claim to eliminate once every two or three days, or once a week, or even less frequently. Sometimes these bm types are under the impression that they are not constipated because they actually eliminate at least once a day, even though the volume of waste is a mere fraction of what they ate the day before and looks more like rabbit droppings than human fecal matter. These people need to understand about *transit time*. Transit time refers to the amount of time it takes your body to digest the foods you eat, absorb and assimilate the nutrients from those foods and then eliminate the rest as waste. Normal healthy transit time is right around 24 hours. Transit time is "clocked" from the time you finish any meal, until that meal shows up in your toilet bowel as waste. There is a simple way to test your transit time (page 60). It is not critical that you know your transit time in order to heal your problem, but it makes for a great story after you do. I have people who tell me they are not constipated, but when they check their transit time they are shocked to discover three and four and five day transit times instead of the normal 24 hour period. What is your transit time?

Type 2 The loose, mushy, spasmodic, irritated, diarrhea-like bowel movement. This person often feels an unstoppable urgency to go and is prone to accidents of the most embarrassing kind (fecal incontinence).

This type of bowel problem results in one such movement per day, to as many as 20 (usually urgent) trips to the bathroom per day (or more). You already read about the young man with ulcerative colitis who missed his college graduation ceremony because he could not be away from the toilet for more than 30 minutes at a time in the personal stories section of Section One. That's not just sad, it's tragic. But you may already know how tragic this is from your own direct personal experience or from someone you love.

Type 3 Combinations of Types 1 and 2 above. There is no set pattern for your bowel movements. There is no way to consistently predict what is going to happen on any given day. Sometimes you are constipated and sometimes you have loose, mushy bowel movements. Sometimes you have something in between. Sometimes you have both, during the same bowel movement. Your bowel movements are always unpredictable. The only consistent thing about your bowel movements is their consistent unpredictability.

All three types of people (and their bowel movements) need to follow the first five steps of my *Intestinal Regeneration Program* as described below in the *What to Do Next* section. As you begin to implement these instructions, I will make very important and clear distinctions between the three major types of bowel movement problems and exactly how each type is to proceed with its (your) *Intestinal Regeneration Program*.

🍇 The Three Phases of Your Intestinal Regeneration Program

Phase One of your *Intestinal Regeneration Program* will provide you with relief from whatever troubling symptoms you are currently experiencing. The time it takes to experience this relief could be several days or several weeks. It depends upon how quickly you are able to get all the steps of the progam working together synergistically and how consistently you practice them. It also depends on the severity of your condition and symptoms. In most cases, it is only a matter of several days before the vast majority of my clients tell me that they are starting to feel better. Whatever time it takes, it is remarkably little time compared to the amount of time you have already suffered. So, please be patient, and keep implementing the suggestions that make up this program.

Once your symptoms are gone, you will need to exercise special care and vigilance. You will need to maintain a certain amount of discipline and commitment while your digestive system is stabilizing and getting ready for Phase Two of your natural healing process. The time period for Phase Two of your natural healing process will be at least several weeks, and most likely several months. The biggest danger and temptation during Phase Two of your *Intestinal Regeneration Program* is to equate the lack of uncomfortable symptoms with complete and total healing. Nothing could be further from the truth. For every year you have been symptomatic, you should expect at least a month or two or three in the Phase Two recovery and stabilization period. If you have been symptomatic for five years for example, your Phase Two recovery period will be at least five months and perhaps as long as fifteen months. This is still miraculous from any common sense point of view, so again, be patient and show some appreciation for the natural healing process.

The second phase of your *Intestinal Regeneration Program* will provide your body the opportunity to physically rebuild your entire digestive system: cell by cell, section by section, organ by organ. You will know you have successfully graduated into Phase Two when you are able to effectively digest and tolerate a wider variety of foods and beverages with significantly greater comfort and ease. You may experience occasional discomfort during Phase Two, but it will most likely be mild, unless you really overdo it.

However, as a result of putting yourself correctly through this program, you will understand what you did to create the discomfort and what you can do in the future to prevent it. *It will always be your choice to invite your symptoms back again or not.*

The third and final phase of your *Intestinal Regeneration Program* will find you experiencing a level of health and vitality you may never have experienced before. The best way to describe this level of intestinal regeneration and overall health and well being would be: *the experience of total dietary freedom.*

I want you to be free to eat whatever you want to eat whenever you want to eat it. Imagine that.

Any dietary or lifestyle *restrictions* that you may encounter during the first two phases of your *Intestinal Regeneration Program* are temporary. How temporary? Whatever it takes! Usually a few months to several months time is all that is required. You need to learn how to restore normal functioning to your digestive system. In order to do that, you need to quiet things down, calm things down and settle things down inside your digestive system. In order to do that, you need to select foods and beverages that complement normal intestinal functioning and you need to avoid (like the plague) any foods and beverages that may be insulting to normal intestinal functioning. Just remember that any food and beverage restrictions are temporary and necessary to restore normal functioning to your digestive system and you will do just fine, like the thousands of people who have come before you. Rome was not built in a day. Be patient. This is common sense.

To me, the very best definition of health is this: *the ability to digest anything.* Imagine that.

When you achieve the goal of *total dietary freedom* is completely up to you. My job is to teach you the most important fundamentals and provide you with a reliable map and compass for the journey ahead.

Section 2 - Getting Started

Getting to the destination of *total dietary freedom* is an adventure unique to each of us, and no one else can take us *all the way there*. We make the way ourselves, one step at a time, one day at a time, one decision at a time.

Now that we have caught a glimpse of the future, let's return to the reality of the situation today. Don't worry about Phase Three. Don't worry about Phase Two. Just focus on integrating the suggestions found in Steps 1-6 described below. This is Phase One.

The journey of a thousand miles begins with the first step.

Let's get started!

Section 2 - Getting Started

Phase One:
What to Do Next

Step 1: Exercise Mindfulness
Directions begin on page 119.
Step 2: Start doing the watercure right away.
Directions begin on page 120.
Step 3: Order your colon cleanse products.
Directions begin on page 131.
Step 4: Order your digestive system supplements.
Directions begin on page 132.
Step 5: Start your new food program.
Directions begin on page 141.
Step 6: Read, The Habits of Functional Nutrition.
Directions begin on page 157.

Exercise Mindfulness

Mindfulness is another word for self-awareness. The most important step we can take and the most important habit we can develop is mindfulness. Pay more attention to everything that affects your life and health but pay more attention in particular to what you eat and how you eat and when you eat and why you eat. Slow down. Observe. Make connections. Connect the dots. Healing ourselves starts with mindfulness and mindfulness is the best form of common sense and wisdom we possess, but it doesn't happen automatically. We must turn it on. We must actively choose, purposefully pursue and consciously cultivate the habit of mindfulness.

Section 2 - Getting Started

The Watercure Recipe

This is the basic recipe as taught by F.Batmanghelidj MD in his book: *Your Body's Many Cries for Water* (and his other books) and on his website: www.watercure.com I urge you to go to this site and to read his books for additional information about the role of proper daily hydration and health and for in-depth scientific analysis and explanations that are beyond the scope of this book. All bowel types (1, 2, and 3) need to do the watercure exactly as described below. If you find any discrepancies or contradictions in any information you find outside of this book, please go to my website and check the FAQ section. If you do not find your answers there, by all means post your question or concern on my website: www.healingdigestiveillness.com.

Sadly, Dr. B. passed away in the fall of 2004. He was 72 years old. He died from the complications of pneumonia. More information is available on his website. Fortunately for me, I had one last opportunity to speak with him just a few weeks before he died. He telephoned me one day in November 2004, out of the blue and greeted me with the following: "Hello Russell, you'll never guess who this is!" His voice was unmistakable. I said; "Of course I know who this is. It's Dr.B! What a pleasant surprise, how can I help you today?" He went on to tell me a story about how he had recently moved his office from one location to another, and when he moved his desk, he found a letter that I had written to him in the spring of 2002. This had been the last time we had been in touch with each other. He apologized to me, because he had intended to publish my letter in one of his books. He was calling on this day, to say that he was in the final editing stages of his newest book, (**Obesity, Cancer, Depression**) and he wanted my permission to include my letter in this new one. I said yes. Here is a copy of that letter:

The Center for Functional Nutrition
514 Amherst Road, South Hadley, MA 01075
413-536-3322

F. Batmanghelidj, MD
Global Health Solutions, Inc.
PO Box 3189   Falls Church, VA   22043

April 23, 2002
Dear Dr. B,
This is a letter that is long overdue!

Since 1973, when I was incorrectly diagnosed with colon cancer and then ineffectively treated for ulcerative colitis, I have been on a quest to discover the fundamental connections between our nutritional choices and our health. Scientific studies, though often helpful, should never be a replacement for our own direct personal experiences. Thank you for encouraging people to take more responsibility for their own health and well-being by taking actions that truly nourish them best.

In my own experience, I was shocked to discover how little I understood about the cause and effect relationships between states of *chronic unintentional dehydration* and disease. Even in my natural healing classes I had been advised to *eat when you're hungry and drink when you're thirsty*. I had been taught that there was enough water content in the cooked whole-grains, steamed vegetables, and fresh fruits that I was eating and that extra water was rarely necessary. I was taught that drinking water would dilute and render ineffective the digestive juices. I was taught that drinking water would weaken my kidneys. How incorrect all that advice turned out to be! Although I had always made a point of drinking only fresh spring water or purified tap water, there were many years of my life that I rarely drank more than one or two glasses of water per day. For most of the past thirty years, I have weighed an average of two hundred pounds. So you can see that my daily water intake had been woefully inadequate for a very long time.

Section 2 - Getting Started

My body was constantly crying out to me for water and salt, but I did not know how to interpret these messages. Irritable bowel, chronic fatigue, dry skin, days of acute anxiety, weeks of constant depression and periodic kidney stones were all signals of thirst and chronic dehydration that I missed for many, many years. More importantly, because of my own ignorance of the role of proper daily hydration and health, I was unable to pass this vital information on to others. Fortunately, all of that changed about five years ago.

In the middle of one of the worst episodes of acute anxiety and constant depression in my life, someone handed me your first book: *Your Body's Many Cries for Water*. After reading chapter 5 on *Stress and Depression*, I had the thought: "Why haven't I ever read or heard anything about this before?" Your explanations all made perfect sense. A few days later I phoned your office and spoke to you in person. You simply advised me to begin measuring the inflow of water and the outflow of urine, and to consume half my body weight in ounces of water with salt, daily. Thus began one of the most helpful and important learning experiences of my life.

Following your sage advice, it took a mere *fourteen days* for my body to rid itself of the state of anxiety and depression that I had been suffering from for almost two months.

Remember, that I had been suffering from periodic (and medically unexplainable) bouts of anxiety and depression for over *twenty years*. In the previous three years, I had also started to experience the excruciating pain of kidney stones, which came upon me like clockwork in the late summers of 1994, 1995 and 1996 (all caused by dehydration!).

Since first learning about *the watercure* in March 1997, I have not had one relapse of anxiety or depression. I have not had another kidney stone attack either. I know with absolute confidence and certainty that both of these *medically unexplainable conditions* had their origin in my state of chronic unintentional dehydration. As the weeks and months and years roll by, the benefits of proper daily hydration continue to manifest.

Clearly, there exists no more powerful medicine on earth than simple water and salt! Clearly, the easiest thing each one of us can do every single day to ensure the highest quality of health inside our own bodies is to maintain proper hydration levels within the cells, organs and systems by drinking the correct amounts of water with salt. In the hierarchy of effective health solutions, nothing is more important than water with salt. The *water-cure* is health solution number one!

I have tried many natural, alternative and holistic health suggestions for over thirty years now, and all of them have worked to one degree or another. Water with salt is the thing that ties them all together. When the body is properly hydrated on a daily basis, every other complementary health habit is enhanced and made more effective. For many people this habit of water with salt is the missing piece of the puzzle in their long search for effective health solutions. In my work with clients in my nutrition counseling practice, it is the very first thing I teach them.

Thank you for your pioneering work in educating the world about the role of proper daily hydration and health. I am committed to helping you get the word out. The watercure is not only vital; it's transformational. Ignorance truly is the cause of all human suffering. Education, of the kind you continue to provide us all, is the very best medicine we have.

Sincerely,

Russell Mariani

May the good Dr. B. rest in peace in that eternal home beyond this life. May the rest of us work diligently and tirelessly, as he did, until every one we know and love becomes properly educated and informed about this life-changing information and advice.

Since first learning about this essential piece of the health and nutrition puzzle back in 1997, I have practiced this *most fundamental of complementary habits* every single day. I have recommended it to many others, and I have learned a few things to make it even more effective. I discussed these things with Dr. B in our last conversation. The bottom line is this: it works. Chronic unintentional dehydration is at the root cause of every symptom of imbalance we humans suffer from. 65–85% of every cell in our body is composed of water, and when there is draught at any level, basic functions are impaired. It is very likely that some or all of the symptoms you are currently suffering from have part of their root cause in a condition of chronic unintentional dehydration, especially constipation! Here's how the watercure works!

The Watercure Recipe

1. The water you drink must be free of all impurities. If you do not have an effective point-of-use home water purifier, let me know and I will send you information about the unit I have been using and

recommending for over 25 years. It converts your tap water into purified water 99.99% free of all impurities for less than ten cents a gallon. Do not drink tap water. Do not use an inferior quality faucet filter as they often make your water quality worse not better. If you must, go to your local health food store and buy the bottled water they recommend. But the use of any bottled water should be temporary.

2. The water you drink must be warm. Not hot, not cold, warm. The best temperature varies from person to person based on body type, metabolism, and current state of health. Room temperature may be too cool because water, standing alone, will always want to return to its original temperature. For most people starting out and for all people with an inflammatory condition during phase one, body temperature water is best. Our normal internal body temperature is 98.6 degrees. Your body works very hard to maintain this internal temperature. When you are sick, it takes extra energy and extra nutrients to maintain homeostasis, including your internal body temperature.

3. The water you drink must contain salt. Sea salt is best. Celtic sea salt is the best sea salt. One quarter teaspoon of salt per one quart of drinking water. One quart is 32 ounces. The Celtic sea salt from the Grain and Salt Society is now available in many retail stores. You can also phone them at 1-800-867-7258. (www.celticseasalt.com) I use and recommend the Light Gray Salt. The reason for adding the salt to your water is to aid the process of absorption and assimilation of the water molecules into your blood and into your cells. The presence of the salt also has an alkalinizing effect which is conducive to the natural healing process. If you cannot handle the taste of one quarter teaspoon of salt per quart of water, don't worry. Just start with a smaller amount, even if that smaller amount is one grain of salt per quart of water. Then just build up gradually over days and weeks until you reach compliant levels. Most people have some difficulty when first drinking intentionally salted water. These same people also report that they prefer the salted water once they get used to it and once they experience the profound benefits of proper daily hydration. There is more information in the next few paragraphs below under the heading: **Why is Proper Daily Hydration So Important?**

4. Drink your salted water throughout the entire day. Sip your water. Don't drink 6-8 oz at a time. Drink 1-2 oz at a time. Go slowly. Sip water throughout the day. Be gentle. Try not to drink too fast or drink too much at any one time. Try to space it out evenly

throughout the day. If you have a history of incontinence, other bladder problems, frequent bladder and urinary tract infections, or you are concerned about the increased amount of water you will be drinking…relax. This isn't something I am telling you about because it sounded like a good idea. This is a powerful solution to all kinds of problems. I have witnessed this in my own life and in the lives of my clients during the last seventeen years. As your kidneys and bladder become properly re-hydrated their normal functions will get better not worse and any associated problems in these areas will get better, not worse. Just follow these directions precisely. Be patient. Go slow but steady.

5. Drink at least 16-24-32oz of warm salted water within the first hour of waking up each day. Try to wake up within an hour of sunrise if at all possible. Our body co-exists in a natural symbiotic relationship with the seasons and the tides and the rising and setting of the sun. Natural healing co-exists in harmony with the forces at work in the natural world. These same forces are at work inside our bodies. Each morning our body is the most dehydrated, the most acidic and the most toxic. This habit of starting each day by consuming 16-24-32oz of salted water within the first hour of waking up is a very important key to getting and maintaining the very best results possible from the watercure. If you weigh less than 150 pounds, then you can start your day with 16-24 ounces of salted water. (Yes, children too.) Use common sense. If this seems like too much for you, start with a smaller amount and build up to compliance levels more gradually.

6. The amount of urine you eliminate should be equal to the amount of water you drink each day. It may take several days but not usually more than several weeks to see this balance happening with your body. You've never measured your outflow of urine? Neither had I. Join the club. Hey, we get to do all kinds of strange and curious things in the name of natural healing. The color of the first morning urine can be moderately yellow, but the rest of the urine should be very light yellow to almost clear like the color of lite beer. Dark yellow to orange colored urine is a sure-sign of dehydration and possible kidney stagnation which is not good. If the color of your urine is currently orange or very dark yellow and it does not become significantly lighter within several days of doing the water-cure, you should check with your medical doctor right away.

7. You must consume half your body weight in ounces of water per day, each and every day to recover from the symptoms of long

term, chronic, unintentional dehydration and to prevent it from happening again. Read that rather long sentence again, and then several times after that, for it represents the most important part of the watercure recipe. You must consume the right quality water and you must consume the right amount or quantity of water. I have never been one for "set prescriptions" especially when it comes to our food and beverage intake. Set prescriptions are usually reserved for drugs, not for habits in the world of natural healing. However, there are always exceptions to the rules and this is absolutely one of those exceptional rules.

Please do not underestimate the importance of being consistent with the correct amount of water you need to drink each day. Water and salt in combination promote and restore proper hydration levels within the cells and systems of the body. Proper daily hydration is the most significant biomodulating and homeostatic influence inside the human body. When the body is properly and consistently hydrated, everything else functions better. If you exercise and sweat, consume any diuretic beverages (alcohol, coffee, tea, soda, caffeine), then you will need to consume more water to make up. Your body loses 32 ounces of water each day just from breathing and sleeping and sitting around! If you exert yourself vigorously and sweat profusely, you will need to be very careful to restore proper hydration levels and then maintain proper hydration levels. Half your body weight in ounces of water is therefore, the absolute minimum of water you need each day. But don't over-hydrate yourself either. Find the balance. Find the right amount of water for you given your unique circumstances and conditions.

Let's summarize the steps of the watercure recipe for easier reference and understanding:

1. The water we drink must be free of all impurities. Sip, do not gulp your water.
2. The water we drink must be warm. Body temperature water is best.
3. Every ounce of water you drink must contain the Celtic sea salt for best results.
4. Drink your warm salted water throughout the entire day. Space-it-out. Sip.
5. Drink 16-24-32 oz of warm salted water within the first hour of waking up each day. If you weigh 150 pounds or less, you can try 12-16-24 oz to start the day.

Section 2 - Getting Started

6. The outflow of urine should be equal in volume to the inflow of water. The color of your urine should be very light yellow like the color of lite beer.
7. You must consume half your body weight in ounces of warm salted water every day. If you weigh 200 pounds you need to drink 100 ounces of water. It's just this simple.

Why Is Proper Daily Hydration So Important?

You need to understand that your body is likely suffering from a condition of ***chronic unintentional dehydration.*** Remember, I said ***unintentional.***

This is not necessarily the primary cause of your uncomfortable digestive system problems and symptoms, (or other health concerns) but it is a major contributing factor. When this dehydration problem is corrected, your symptoms could disappear altogether. Proper daily hydration is transformational.

You have just read about the seven steps that make up the watercure recipe. You must follow this recipe as described as soon as possible. This means that depending on your unique circumstances and conditions, it might take you three days to make this transition and it might take you three weeks. What matters most is that you get to 100% compliance as soon as you possibly can. Don't rush, but don't procrastinate either.

For the very best results possible, please order some Celtic sea salt right away. For the best prices and how to order, see the information below. Use whatever sea salt you have on hand, or get some at your local health food store, until you get the Celtic sea salt. Some natural food stores are now carrying the Celtic Salt; Whole Foods Market for example. Or order online at www.celticseasalt.com The Celtic sea salt contains many other minerals and trace minerals (over 40) and this allows for better absorption into the cells, better communication between cells and the incalculable therapeutic effects of alkalinizing our blood and lymph. I keep using this term, alkalinizing, but what I really mean is stabilizing our body fluids at their proper pH levels. For example, the pH of human blood must remain constant at 7.35 to 7.45

for optimum health. The pH of ocean water is nearly identical to the pH of human blood. Imagine that.

The primary reason commercial table salt is so bad for us is that it is almost pure sodium chloride. It has been stripped of all other minerals. This kind of salt is not natural at all. It is highly processed and refined. It is even bleached to be white. No wonder it is toxic to the body! Naturally harvested salt from the ocean is gray and moist, not white and dry.

When you use the Celtic sea salt in the correct amounts according to the watercure recipe you will not increase the problems normally associated with the excess use of salt, you will decrease their likelihood of occurrence. This is because of the dramatic qualitative differences between organic quality sea salt and commercial quality highly processed and refined table salt. Use the sea salt. Don't use the commercial table salt. If you are not sure what you should do and have not been convinced by now of the therapeutic value of sea salt, please do not proceed.

I talk to people all the time who claim to drink tons of water. These same people will report astonishing results as soon as they start adding salt per the instructions of the watercure recipe. The combination of water and salt is a powerful natural remedy for all kinds of problems.

The warm salted water we drink is absorbed into our body through the stomach. Follow these suggestions (sipping constantly throughout the day) and you will not feel bloated. Your bladder will get stronger not weaker. Your bladder capacity will increase and if you suffer from the symptoms of frequent urination and/or incontinence, they will subside and eventually disappear altogether. You must drink your water on an empty stomach and before meals. Wait about 20-30 minutes after meals before resuming your water intake or you may dilute your digestive juices, which is not good. Sometimes you need to wait longer. Experiment. You decide.

There is still some debate about this last point but I would rather err on the side of caution and my last 17 years of observations and personal experience. As I have said many times already, when you are feeling healthy and whole and strong again, you will need to take all of my "suggestions" with a grain of salt and mostly rely on your own experimenting to ultimately find out what works best for you. But this advice is for down the road, well into Phase Two or even into Phase Three. In Phase One, it is best to follow my suggestions as described here.

Think of *proper daily hydration* as the foundation of your physical health habits. Everything else you learn and do about *Functional Nutrition* and *Intestinal Regeneration* will be built upon this one simple habit. Everything else you do will work better if you practice this habit of proper daily hydration effectively. And everything else you do will work less effectively if you do not practice this daily hydration habit correctly and consistently. A word to the wise is sufficient.

Purchasing Your Celtic Sea Salt from The Grain and Salt Society:

First check out their website: www.celticseasalt.com. There are often introductory specials that will include the best prices. I use and recommend the light-gray Celtic sea salt to begin with. This company has lots of interesting products and information. When you are ready to order, phone them at 800-867-7258 or order online. Also visit www.selinanaturally.com

Supplements to Order

Order Your Colon Cleanse Products

Call the American Botanical Pharmacy at 1-800-437-2362. Tell the Order Operator that you have been referred by me (Russell Mariani) and that you have a **Practitioner Referral** number for your first order. This gets you a 10% discount. That number is: **PR133**. This company is in California.

Tell the Order Operator that you need **4 containers** of **Intestinal Formula #2** (bulk powder unless you prefer capsules; just keep in mind that each dose of IF#2 is 5-10 capsules; some people prefer mixing the powder with water rather than swallowing that many capsules several times a day. The choice is yours.) and **1 large bottle of Intestinal Formula #1** (regular strength) and **2 containers of a product called Herbal-Mucil Plus**(this is in bulk-powder form). From now on, when I refer to these three products I will use the following abbreviations: **IF#1** (Intestinal Formula #1) **IF#2** (Intestinal Formula #2) and **hm+** (HerbalMucil Plus) **I also want you to order 2 bottles of a product called: Digestive Tonic.** Digestive Tonic is formulated to address and relieve any symptoms in the stomach. And at night, it helps to settle the stomach, allowing for easier sleep. This is a one time purchase not a monthly purchase. Some products in this group may need to be reordered depending on your condition, symptoms and progress.

If you have any trouble whatsoever placing this order, phone Megan Moore in our office here at 413-536-3322. She will be happy to help.

Section 2 - Getting Started

Order your Digestive System Supplements

This company is in Oregon, which is Pacific Standard Time zone; PST. Their toll-free number is: 1-800-800-1300. It is best to order these products via telephone and speak directly with a Phone Order Operator. (don't order online) **It is very important that you follow my phone ordering instructions below: Tell the New Earth Order Operator:**

1. You would like to place your first order as a **Preferred Customer**:

2. Your **Sponsor** is Russell Mariani and his New Earth ID number is: 1032997

3. You want to order the following products: **three (3) boxes of Essentials** and **two (2) bottles** of a product called: **Spectrabiotic,**

Each packet of **Essentials** contains two capsules of blue green algae, one capsule of digestive enzymes and two capsules of probiotics. The Blue Green Algae is your full spectrum multi-vitamin, multi-mineral, multi-micronutrient supplement. **Spectrabiotic** is a full spectrum probiotic.

This next paragraph is VERY important: How to set up your monthly AutoShip with New Earth.

Before you complete your first Phone Order Transaction with New Earth, I need you to set yourself up for a monthly automatic order which is called an **AutoShip** order. This will guarantee that you do not run out of product within the first 30 days of your program. Set up your **AutoShip** order to take place **24 days from today... and then monthly 24 days from that day.** (Just make sure your products arrive within 30 calendar days of each order so you don't run out. This is very important.) All AutoShip orders are set up ONLY on the following calendar days: 1st, 5th, 10th, 15th and 20th.

Set up a monthly AutoShip Order for **3 Boxes of Essentials**. There are no fees attached to this **AutoShip** service and as a Preferred Client or Preferred Customer you will be paying Wholesale prices. Plan on consuming these products per the guidelines below for three to six months for best results.

If you have any trouble whatsoever placing this order, phone Megan Moore in our office here at 413-536-3322. She will be happy to help.

🌰 How to Use the Supplements

Please understand that as simple, safe and effective as my program is, your condition has many moving parts and not everyone is going to be immediately successful in adapting ideas from a book or ebook or website and making everything work smoothly without a few bumps along the way. Mistakes and misjudgements are inevitable. So be patient with yourself if you are doing this on your own. Being proactive and exercising common sense are your most important habits in your successful healing journey.

Healing ourselves is a unique, individual and very organic process. Each body adjusts to change in slightly different ways. It's really impossible for any book or website to make it easy for everyone to be able to heal themselves 100% of the time. If it was that easy, that book and set of guidelines would already have been written and everyone would own it, use it and be perfectly healthy.

I have done my very best to explain everything as clearly as I can in this book and the truth is that since it's original publication in 2006 many people have used these guidelines to heal themselves and you can too and you can read those testimonials on my website.

And, if you are in pain or major discomfort and you have been diagnosed with an "official" inflammatory bowel disorder (IBD) like Crohn's or Colitis, or Ulcerative Colitis, or any other Digestive System Disorder like Colonic Inertia, Celiac Disease, Acid Reflux Disease, GERD, Chronic Constipation, Colonic Inertia, Gastroparesis, etc please consider becoming a client so that I can walk you through the entire program step by step by step.

Specific Product Usage Guidelines

New Earth Products

I have been using and recommending the products from this company since 1987. Originally called Cell Tech, from 1983 to 2006, then SimpleXity Health from 2006 to 2013, and now called New Earth. The name of the company and various products may change, but the transformational quality of these wild-grown, plant-based, superfood supplements continue to stand head and shoulders above the rest.

The Three Types of Digestive System Supplements You Need

You need to provide a full spectrum of micro-nutrients, so that every cell of your digestive system can repair itself, detoxify itself, nourish itself, and regenerate itself. You need to provide supplemental digestive enzymes to make sure that all the food you eat gets broken down and turned into liquid for easier absorption and assimilation. Lastly, you need to provide the very best probiotic materials in order to replace all the bad bacteria in your gut with good bacteria. For these reasons, the wild blue green algae, the digestive enzymes and the probiotic products from the New Earth company have been core components of my Intestinal Regeneration Program for over 25 years.

SBGA contains vitamins, minerals, trace-minerals, all twenty amino acids, phyto-nutrients, anti-oxidants, active enzymes, pigments, essential fatty acids, and much more. And it is 100% certified organic. Super Blue Green Algae contains over 80 different micro-nutrients.

Gram for gram it is the most nutrient-rich superfood ever discovered. It contains all these essential micro-nutrients in a balanced and highly absorbable whole food form.

Supplemental digestive enzymes break down our foods into their tiniest components in order to make it possible for their absorption and assimilation into our bloodstream through the villi and microvilli of the small intestine. Enyzmes in general and digestive enzymes in particular provide many benefits as an integral part of the normal functioning of our body. Here is a short list: purify the blood and lymph, strengthen the immune system, break down fats, lower cholesterol, help in weight loss, improve skin quality, help cleanse the colon, increase mental clarity, focus, and memory, and improve sleep.

Supplemental Probiotics are not optional for regaining and maintaining normal digestive system health. They are mandatory. Traditional peoples got their probiotics through certain fermented foods, like pickles, yogurt, kefir, sauerkraut, and miso. Many of these foods are available again in most whole food supermarkets. For most people, the easiest way to get them working inside your gut again is in supplement form. Probiotics maintain the health of the mucous lining of the digestive system. They service and protect the billions of villi and micro-villi and help to maintain the pH of the entire digestive system. Probiotics produce vitamins (including all the B-vitamins), and antibiotics, and protect our immune system.

For more information and comprehensive product descriptions and ingredient listings go to; www.newearth.com

New Earth Products Usage Guidelines

Typically I have clients consume one packet of Essentials before each major meal. Most people do fine starting off with three packets of Essentials on day one. Some people find it more effective to build up gradually to these amounts. Spectrabiotic is used AFTER the completion of the colon cleanse. Wild Blue Green Blend is used throughout the program starting with one level teaspoon mixed in a small amount of water in a jar with a lid, per day. Depending on a person's level of micronutrient deficiency, more Wild Blue Green Blend can be used. Super Blue Green Algae is the world's number one superfood containing more necessary and essential micronutrients, gram for gram, than any other food plant on planet earth. This means that increasing the amount of Super Blue Green Algae from one gram a day to three or five grams a day or more, has proven to be totally safe and totally effective in many programs.

If you do not like the Wild Blue Green Blend powder, you can purchase equal amounts of the products Wild Blue Green Body and Wild Blue Green Mind. These are the two forms of Super Blue Green Algae that come in tablet or capsule form.

When your colon cleanse is complete you can start taking two capsules of Spectrabiotic with your Essentials, before meals. Two bottles of Spectrabiotic is usually enough but in some cases of really extensive dysbiosis 4 bottles has been more effective.

Some people have found that purchasing the three core New Earth products of Blue Green Algae, Digestive Enzymes and Probiotics separately (separate bottles) allows them more flexibility for experimentation. For example, there is one capsule of digestive enzymes in each packet of the Essentials, but some people with upper GI problems report doing much better with 4-8 capsules of Digestive Enzymes before meals. The same has been found to be true with Probiotics and of course the blue green algae.

It's not always true that more is better, but sometimes it is, especially when we are in the process of recovering our health; especially in phase one and phase two.

For information about New Earth products please contact Megan Moore at meganmoore3@verizon.net or phone her at 413-536-3322.

The American Botanical Pharmacy

Comprehensive product descriptions including comprehensive ingredients listings for each of the products listed below can be found at www.herbdoc.com

I recommend the use of the product called **Digestive Tonic** for all upper GI problems(GERD, Acid Reflux, heartburn, etc) and for clients to simply follow the usage guidelines on the label.

HerbalMucil Plus (from now on referred to as hm+) is a wonderful product that helps to make for easier flowing bms for people with mild constipation or just sluggish and incomplete bms. Hm+ is also very helpful at any point of one's colon cleanse when it becomes difficult to determine the correct amount of IF#1 each day.

Sometimes it feels like 4IF#1 is too much, but taking 3IF#1 is just not enough. In this situation, where 3IF#1 is not enough to produce the desired bm result, just adding one dose of hm+ per day will often make the difference. For best results follow the preparation and consumption guidelines for hm+ below.

Section 2 - Getting Started

HerbalMucil Plus Instructions

Find a clean, empty glass or plastic jar with a lid. An 8oz mason jar does nicely or an empty peanut butter jar; or any glass or plastic jar with a lid. Add 4-6 oz of your normal body temperature salted drinking water to the empty jar. Start out with a level teaspoon per dose. Everyone is different and every condition is different. Typically hm+ is taken once a day but some people have found best results taking it two or three times a day. Doses can range from half a teaspoon to a heaping teaspoon to a level tablespoon to a heaping or rounded tablespoon. Experiment to find out what works best for you and your condition.

Add the hm+ to the water and very quickly put the lid on and even more quickly shake it up vigorously for a count of five seconds, then remove the lid and drink it all down quickly; and do all this without rushing.

Yes, you can add more water to help remix it and make it less thick and to wash it down. You may want to add some more water to the jar to make sure you get all the hm+ that may stick to the sides, etc.

This is a very light remedy made mostly from psyllium husks and seeds and sits very easily and gently in your stomach. It will help you sleep. It is best to take this just before going to bed, as it will then work through your system while you are sleeping and you will notice better bms in the morning.

It seems to take about 6-8 hours to work its way through your entire digestive system, so keep that in mind if you take it at other times of the day.

The herbalmucil plus is helpful for anyone with a sluggish colon at any level; from mild occasional constipation to extreme colonic inertia. It is made from highest quality 100% organic herbs. It is totally safe and very effective.

The following information is from the American Botanical Pharmacy catalog and can also be found at www.herbdoc.com

"HerbalMucil Plus holds more water in suspension in your food waste so it doesn't get dried out or become too hard in your colon. This added liquid makes it very easy to have effortless normal bms. HerbalMucil Plus is also very mucilaginous or "slippery" which also aids in an easier elimination.

HerbalMucil Plus is loaded with pure plant fiber which also contributes to a very comfortable, easy, more natural bm. HerbalMucil Plus contains whole leaf aloe vera cactus which adds a mild extra push to help you eliminate more easily and completely. The HerbalMucil

Plus powder has a very neutral taste, but when it gets into your colon, it forms a fibrous, mucilaginous gel that gives you easy, magical bowel movements!"

Intestinal Formula #1 (from now on referred to as IF#1) contains stool softeners and cathartic and purgative herbs. IF#1 is for people suffering from constipation and colonic inertia. IF#1 is almost always taken on a full stomach immediately after the evening meal or the last meal of the day. Start with one capsule only and increase by one capsule per day until the desired result is achieved. Desired results means that you are having one or two or three at the most, soft formed bms per day preferably within the first few hours each day or within an hour of every major meal. Bms should come out easily, effortlessly, without straining. You should feel empty and complete after the last bm each day. Your colon transit time should be a minimum of 18 hours and a maximum of 30 hours. 24 hours is ideal.

Obviously, if you are suffering from an inflammatory bowel problem and your current condition is defined by loose, urgent, frequent bms; do NOT take the IF#1.

Once your bms flow easily, then you can begin to add the **Intestinal Formula #2** (from now on referred to as IF#2) to your routine. If your condition is defined by loose, urgent, frequent bms you can start your colon cleanse by taking IF#2. One dose is ten capsules or a rounded tablespoon of the powder. Start with four doses a day. Separate each dose by 4-5 hours. Most people find the best times to take IF#2 to be at breakfast time, lunch time, dinner time and before bed. If you need to take 5 or 6 or 7 doses within a 24 hour period to slow things down and get bms formed, do it. It is perfectly safe to do so.

Mix the IF#2 powder in the very same way you were instructed to mix the hm+ in the section above.

If your condition when starting this program was defined by constipation, colonic inertia and sluggish bms, then introduce the IF#2 more gradually. You can begin with half doses of the IF#2 which is 5 capsules or a level teaspoon of the powder. Start with one dose per day and adjust the amount of IF#1 and hm+ accordingly to maintain easy flowing soft formed bms. Build up to three or four doses of IF#2 per day until you have consumed four bottles or containers of IF#2.

If you are doing the watercure as your means of regaining and maintaining proper daily hydration levels, (and you should be) than simply take as much water as you need to easily consume each dose of IF#2. Instructions on the IF#2 label may suggest that you need to drink 16oz of water per dose. I have found over many years that this is not necessary **if you are doing the watercure**. Please understand however that being properly hydrated is mandatory not optional if you are to get the best results from your colon cleanse and reconditioning program.

If you are not properly hydrated, according to the guidelines of the watercure recipe, do not take any Intestinal Formula #2. Do not attempt any of these products or procedures unless you are properly hydrated first.

Unlike IF#1, which is best taken once a day on a full stomach after the evening meal, when you take the IF#2 is totally up to you. Empty stomach, full stomach, before meals, during meals, after meals, in between meals; it doesn't matter. It only matters what feels comfortable to you and that when you are taking multiple doses that you separate each dose by 4-5 hours.

Typically I have my clients consume four containers of IF#2 to make sure that both the small and large intestines have been thoroughly cleansed and detoxified over a 4-5 week period. Sometimes longer depending on circumstances.

Typically after two or three days on full doses of IF#2 the bms will turn black due to the activated charcoal ingredient in the IF#2. So be prepared for that. After a day or two of blackish bms, the bms often turn green; a cooked spinach color green; and this is the physical evidence of the removal of the bad bacteria and all other organisms living in your gut. A major purpose of the intestinal cleanse is to remove all the pathological organisms in the gut (which are causing most if not all of your symptoms) and replace these organisms with healthy bacteria; the probiotics. Typically, if you have never done this kind of colon cleansing and reconditioning before, your "cleanse" is going to last a minimum of 21 days. Most people find that they are completing this part of their program within a 28-35 day window. And some people need longer than this.

If you are attempting to do all this on your own and you are NOT getting the results you desire, please consider contacting me directly and consider becoming a client and let me walk you through the process step by step by step. You can phone me any time during the day at 413-536-0275 or email russellmariani@verizon.net

To summarize:

All parts of this program work together synergistically to bring the normal functions of your digestive and eliminative systems back to normal. It is not the action or result of any one part of the program that produces results. It's the synergistic relationship of all the parts working together that produces the best results. Your goal is to restore normal functioning to your digestive system. Your chances of achieving this goal increase dramatically to the degree you bring mindfulness to everything you do, consistency in all your actions and common sense to determine if you are on course or whether you need more assistance to achieve your goal.

Bring mindfulness to your life in general and your diet in particular. Be and become more proactive in your own self-care. Find and do the things that nourish you best. Pay attention to your habits. No habit has a neutral impact on your digestive health. It's not just what you are eating that makes the difference but why you are eating what you are eating, when, where and how you eat as well.

Do not be distracted when eating. Put on beautiful music. Create a peaceful environment when you consume your meals. Relax. Slow down. Sit down. Chew each mouthful thoroughly. Do not overeat. Do not starve yourself either. Eat more of your food earlier in the day. Eat less food later in the day. Do not snack after your evening meal. Allow at least three hours after your last meal of the day before going to bed and becoming horizontal.

Make sure you are properly hydrated from this day forward. There is no single habit more important than proper daily hydration, other than proper sleep and rest. No one can heal themselves from any disorder or dis-ease without proper sleep and rest. Make sure you exercise your body moderately every single day. You don't have to be a marathon runner or an fitness champion. Walking for 20 minutes at a time for two or three times a day may be all the exercise you need.

You will get well to the degree you find and do the things that nourish you best while you become more proactive in your own self-care.

Section 2 - Getting Started

🌰 Your New Food Program: Phase One Foods Simplified

Your New Food Program will consist of mostly delicious, nutritious organic quality whole foods. Cooked whole grains, cooked vegetables, soups and condiments, and small amounts of animal protein all in balance and proportion to each other. Recipes will be provided. Here is an overview.

Cooked Whole Grains

Cooked Whole Grains have been the single most important staple food in the human diet for at least the past 5,000 years. Nothing fancy here, just plain boiled rice is all you need to make. You do NOT have to make rice (or oats, or barley or millet or buckwheat) daily.

Plan your week and set aside time to make your whole grains twice a week. Two cups of rice, 4-5 cups of water, a pinch of sea salt; bring to a boil, cook until all the water is gone and voila…it doesn't have to be any more complicated than this. Always make sure you wash and rinse any raw whole grain several times before putting it on to cook. To get started purchase only Lundberg Brothers Short Grain Organic Brown Rice (at any Whole Foods Market Store). Follow the guidelines to make cooked whole grains on page 149. Pick the two days of the week that you are going to cook your grains, so that you always have some on hand. It literally takes 5 minutes or less to put a pot of rice on the stove to cook. And while it is cooking you can do other things; like making a pot of soup or steaming some vegetables!

Section 2 - Getting Started

Make a Big Pot of Soup

Making a big pot of vegetable soup or chicken soup is so easy and it's so important. The ingredients can vary or stay the same once you find a combination you really enjoy. Adding a piece of kombu or wakame seaweed to the soup stock adds minerals and trace minerals and a salty flavor. Kombu and wakame seaweeds are very therapeutic foods and aid both digestion and elimination. You can add miso to each individual bowl of soup or not. That's up to you. Miso is another therapeutic food-condiment-supplement that is very alkalinizing in effect, prebiotic in effect and aids in all phases of function; digestion, absorption, assimilation and elimination. You can do this once a week or twice a week.

With these first two (food) steps (cooked whole grains and soup) you will ALWAYS have nutritious, staple; Phase One foods on hand. Foods that nourish and support the regeneration, reconditioning and healing of your entire digestive system.

Make Some Steamed Vegetables Daily

Nothing makes you feel more committed to the task of nourishing yourself with whole foods than cutting and cooking vegetables. When you get into the habit of taking 10-15 minutes every single day to prepare one vegetable and make enough to have on hand as side dishes for the next two days you will never be without best quality food to serve yourself. This is a key to the success of everyone's program. Choose from the list below and on the next page and have at least 10 major healthy vegetables on your shopping list at all times and rotate them and you will be so pleased to discover how important this simple habit is to your overall health and well-being. You can vary the cooking technique of course but simple steaming is all you need to do with these and other core phase one vegetables: broccoli, cauliflower, brussels sprouts, steamed cabbage (yellow, red, green) sautéed onions and bell peppers (red, yellow, green) carrots, parsnips, turnips, buttercup squash, hubbard squash, acorn squash, greens like collards, kale, bok choy, napa, Chinese cabbage, broccoli rabe, etc.

Organic Quality Animal Protein

Organic quality animal protein (even 2-3 bites, even 2-4oz) dramatically extends the energy you get from your meals of soup, whole grains and steamed vegetables, so please keep this in mind. Grilled salmon, poached salmon, baked salmon and other fish like cod, sole, tuna, and even canned fish like sardines, herring, anchovies, tuna; as well as chicken breast, turkey breast, and as conditions improve ground beef, pork chops, lamb chops, sausages, etc. Small amounts of organic quality animal protein can be a part of most people's totally healthy diet. Only in the most extreme conditions of Inflammatory Bowel Disease should animal protein be minimized during Phase One.

When you exercise mindfulness, hydrate effectively, take your supplements correctly and follow these simplified Phase One food and meal ideas and suggestions consistently you will dramatically increase the chances of feeling better faster on the way to total success and healing.

What to eat and what to avoid?

Over the years, from many books, and from many conversations with other educators and practitioners, there is some consensus about what fruits and vegetables are best for regular use, (daily use) occasional use, and what fruits and vegetables are best to avoid completely when you are in the middle of an intestinal flare-up, or inflammatory bowel disorder, like Crohn's Disease, Diverticulitis, Irritable Bowel Syndrome, (IBS) or when there are any symptoms of gas, bloating, diarrhea or abdominal pain. There is one particular family of vegetables called: the nightshade group, that seems to be the most problematic for any person suffering any kind of digestive or intestinal disorder.

What to avoid? The Nightshade Group: Asparagus, eggplant, potatoes, tomatoes, zucchini, spinach, artichoke.

What other fruits and vegetables should be avoided during a flare-up of symptoms? Any hot peppers like jalapenos, Jerusalem artichokes, okra, sweet potatoes, swiss chard, yams, brazil nuts, bananas, cashews, coconuts, dates, figs, grapefruit, kiwi, mangoes, oranges, papaya, pistachios, tangerine, tangelo, lemons, raisins, prunes, dried-fruit of any kind, and the juice made from any fruit.

What to eat?

During Phase One of your recovery period, to re-establish normal intestinal function including normal, regular bowel movements you should have small amounts of miso soup before each meal (not everyone has to do this, only some people) cooked whole grain porridge for breakfast, perhaps some cooked grain at other meals, no processed food of any kind, and a variety of steamed or well cooked vegetables. Root vegetables and cruciferous vegetables are the best, but anything from the following list should be fine. Just make sure you sit down, relax, and chew each mouthful well.

Carrots, turnips, onions, parsnips, daikon, burdock root, (if you can find it) leeks, steamed cabbage (red-purple, green, yellow) scallions, acorn squash, buttercup squash, butternut squash, hubbard squash, broccoli, cauliflower, brussels sprouts, celery, fresh corn, napa cabbage, kale, bok choy, broccoli rabe, chinese cabbage, collard greens, watercress, parsley, mustard greens, red radishes, (and many others).

Most important of all

Mindfulness is most important of all. The awareness and consciousness and attention that you bring to the selection, preparation and consumption of your daily foods is the most important complementary habit you will ever develop. So find and do the things that nourish you best, and all will be well, today and always.

🌰 *Your Old and New Breakfast Routine*

The alarm goes off. You open one startled eye which unconsciously extends a foggy glance into the semi-darkness of your sleeping room. Then both eyes open with reluctance and hesitation and heaviness. You close your eyes and fall back to sleep.

The alarm goes off again. This time, you do not open your eyes, and you do not get up. Your hand stretches out along a familiar route until it grabs hold of your alarm clock and swiftly turns off the alarm. You fall back to sleep in a matter of seconds.

You fly out the door of your apartment and drive down to the nearest Dunkin Donuts. You order a coffee, "Light, no sugar," and two jelly donuts to go.

You reach into the refrigerator and take out the orange juice and pour yourself a cold one. You sit down at the table in your pajamas and robe. You pour cold milk over a bowel of wheat flakes, or corn flakes, or fruit flakes, or chocolate flakes. Maybe you have a piece of toast. Maybe you have a cup of coffee or two before you go. You get to the office and have another coffee or two, and perhaps some donuts that Marge brought in.

You walk into the kitchen and head straight for the coffee maker, which has been timed perfectly to provide you with hot coffee at 6 am. The smell of fresh brewed coffee fills the air. You sip it slowly, surely, engagingly. You stare at the sky-blue tiles above your microwave. You may have two or three cups of coffee before you head off to work. You don't eat anything else.

You walk into the kitchen, open up the freezer, take out some frozen waffles, and pop two into the toaster or toaster oven. You pour artificial maple syrup on top of the waffles. You wash it all down with orange juice. You grab a coffee at the convenience store where you pick up a newspaper on your way to work.

You drive to McDonald's and pick up an Egg McMuffin or two and a coke.

You stop at the Bluebonnet Diner to meet your friend, Danny. You have orange juice, coffee, two-eggs-over-easy, three strips of bacon, home fries, and whole wheat toast.

You juice three large apples, two oranges, and a bunch of purple grapes. You throw in some yogurt and hit *blend*: instant smoothie. You drink it down and head for work.

You sit down to a bowl of organic freshly toasted granola, with slivered almonds and raisins. You add some sliced fruit and top it off with your favorite yogurt or soymilk.

You tear open a package of some protein powder and blend it with orange juice, drink it down, and head off to work.

You boil some water and pour it over some instant oatmeal. You sprinkle your oatmeal with brown sugar and help to wash it down with some green tea.

All of the above scenarios are common American breakfasts experienced by my clients during the past few years, *before* we started working together. Not one of these breakfast scenarios is conducive to digestive system health during Phase One of your *Intestinal Regeneration Program*.

Remember that I did not say forever. I said these breakfast choices were not conducive to digestive system health *during* Phase One. Let me try to explain.

Even though we sleep each night for six or eight hours (more or less), our body is never totally at rest. Digestion, absorption and assimilation of our foods and beverages go on for hours after we finish our last meal of the day, or last snack of the day. Every cell in our body is desperately looking for the micronutrients in our blood and lymph that they will need in order to function normally for the next 24 hours. Every cell in our body is purging itself of simple metabolic toxins and other hazardous materials. Every cell is looking for any damage that occurred during the day and making any necessary repairs. Every ounce of available water is completely used up in these processes, including the movement of fecal waste into our colon.

These activities all require energy. This energy comes from the food we eat and the beverages we drink. But very little of this energy gets manufactured and dispersed from a weak and impaired digestive system.

One definition of insanity is simply this: to do the same thing over and over again while expecting a different result to occur.

In the wee small hours of the morning, your digestive system is dreaming a dream. It is dreaming and hoping that you will wake up in a few hours and prepare a breakfast unlike anything you have ever made before: a breakfast that will be nutritious and easy to digest; a breakfast that will not create the reactions of belching and bloating and gas; a breakfast that will move through your stomach and intestines, attracting and gathering all the undigested bits of food matter along with it from the day before; a breakfast that will enhance the effectiveness of your colon cleanse; a breakfast that will complement the effectiveness of the watercure, and your other supplements; a breakfast that will contribute to the formation of an ideal bowel movement; a breakfast that will settle things down and calm things down along the thirty foot length of your entire digestive system; a breakfast that will let the healing begin.

What is this miraculous breakfast food you ask? Porridge. Yes, porridge.

Most people have never had a bowl of cooked, whole grain porridge, but they think they have. Commercial cereal makers bombard us each day with the benefits of their *"whole grain"* cereal products but they never make the distinction between true whole grains and processed grains. Processed grains are whole grains that have been cut or rolled or crushed into flour and then reconstituted into flakes, puffs, clusters, crackers, granola, etc. These processed breakfast cereals take up entire aisles in our supermarkets. Without exception they are all useless as therapeutic agents (for the purposes of intestinal regeneration), even if they are organic. Products made from processed grains are among the most insulting and most harmful to anyone with digestive system problems. Please avoid them all during Phase One of your *Intestinal Regeneration Program.*

Most people think that oatmeal is a whole grain cereal, but it is not. Oatmeal is useless as a therapeutic food, especially for anyone with digestive system problems. Oatmeal is made from rolled oats, which is a process that strips the whole oat of its vital life-force and full nutrient potency. As a child, I used to make homemade glue with my brothers and sister by mixing water with rolled oats. It does the same thing in our intestines. All processed grain products do the same thing in our intestines, so we should avoid them. We must absolutely avoid these processed grain products during Phase One of our *Intestinal Regeneration Program.*

All whole grains are seeds. You can take a grain of rice or oats or barley and put it in a small container of fertile soil and within a few days, it will sprout. The emerging sprout is called a grass. You can grow wheat grass, barley grass, rice grass, oat grass. These sprouted grasses are very rich in chlorophyll, vitamins, and minerals. Grown and cut and pressed into a pulp, these grasses produce a very nutritious juice. The nutrient content of the sprout or grass or juice depends on the nutrient richness of the soil it grows in. Wheat grass juice is a famous natural healing remedy in use for hundreds of years.

All whole grains are seeds. Agriculture begins with the cultivation of the cereal grains in China, India and in the Middle East. Modern Civilization begins with the cultivation of cereal grains about ten thousand years ago. Cooked whole cereal grains have been the staple food for all human societies experiencing a four-season climate for the last ten thousand years. Cooked whole cereal grains are among the most important and the most nutritious foods on earth. As we have moved away from the habit of cooked whole cereal grains and other traditional staples, we have moved ourselves closer to a pandemic of degenerative diseases unprecedented in the last ten thousand years of our history. It is time to reclaim the value of our oldest and wisest whole foods. Whole grain porridge is one of them. In forty years of constant research and constant experimentation, I have not discovered any single traditional whole food that compares with the therapeutic benefits of cooked whole cereal grains (cooked whole grain porridge).

I once asked my maternal grandfather, William Fulton, for the secret of his health and longevity. He was born in Edinburgh, Scotland in 1903, and came to the United States in his early twenties. He was an apprentice baker in Scotland and worked for the Ward Baking Company in Newark, New Jersey for 40 years. He was responsible for the production of millions of pounds of baked goods over all those years; all processed grain products. He claimed to have never missed a day of work in all that time. I believed him. He did not eat a particularly healthy diet from the day he stepped off the boat until the day he died at the age of 87. He attributed his health and longevity to the first twenty years of his life in Scotland. During those formative years, he ate the traditional diet of his ancestors: oats, peas, beans and barley. This whole grain porridge recipe is a direct link to many of the healthy eating traditions of our ancestors. I hope that in time, we will be able to remember and re-integrate them all.

Whole Grain Porridge: Basic Cooking Instructions

Wash and rinse thoroughly (at least 3 times) one cup of short grain organic quality brown rice (or whole oats or whole barley). I prefer the Lundberg Brothers Organic California Brown Rice, which is available at most health food stores and whole food grocery stores. In a stainless steel pressure cooker or a stainless steel pot, add the one cup of washed and rinsed rice and two cups of purified tap-water (or spring water) and a pinch of organic sea salt. Add a quarter teaspoon of sea salt per one cup of rice. Use the same Celtic Sea Salt as in the watercure recipe. Stir the rice and let it settle so that the rice is evenly distributed around the bottom of the cooking pot. Bring to a boil, then set the pot on a stainless steel flame diffuser and put on a very low flame, to simmer. Simmer for at least one full hour. The longer and slower this cooks, the better the end result will be. Cook the rice (or oats or barley) until all visible water in the pot is gone. If you are using a pressure cooker, you will just have to time it. Don't open your pressure cooker while it is hissing or making any sound whatsoever.

Everyone's stove is slightly different, so you must experiment with the amount of water and the amount of time you cook your whole grains. The goal is to achieve a result that compares with the side of brown rice you would get at a good whole foods restaurant. Each grain of rice (or oats or barley) will have expanded fully, and the skin or shell of each grain will have ruptured. This breaking of the skin of the grain is what releases a starchy material which makes for the cream-like consistency(sometimes but not always). The end result should not be watery, not soup-like, but soft, firm, thick, moist and somewhat sticky. It's very important for the success of your program that you learn to prepare your whole grain porridge correctly. Most of my clients are delighted to discover this recipe and report how delicious it is and how filling and satisfying too. If you get frustrated, locate a whole foods cooking instructor in your area and take some cooking classes right away.

Hippocrates, the father of Western Medicine used barley porridge as a primary remedy. He would recommend hot baths or steam to induce sweating and restrict his patient's food intake for 7 to 14 days to a simple plan of barley porridge and water. No matter what the ailment or complaint, his patients recovered quickly. This recipe for whole grain porridge is the ideal breakfast food for all ages, children, teenagers, young adults, mid-life adults and seniors. It is especially helpful on cold winter mornings. During the summer months it can be allowed to cool down to room temperature and eaten this way, but it should never been eaten cold, as in right out of the refrigerator.

The complex carbohydrates in this whole grain porridge recipe break down very differently in the digestive system than any processed grain product you have used in the past (bread, muffins, bagels, pancakes, flaked cereals, pasta, granola, grits, oatmeal). The complex carbohydrates in whole grain porridge take longer to break down and digest and so its sugars are released more slowly over a longer period of time. This means that you will have more energy for longer periods of time after you eat it; certainly more than any other breakfast cereal or processed-cereal based breakfast food you have had in the past.

For people suffering the most extreme symptoms of Inflammatory Bowel Disease, you may need to limit your food intake during the first few days or weeks of your program to soup, cooked whole grains and some cooked vegetables. Everyone else should feel free to add some animal protein as it was discussed earlier.

You do not have to cook your porridge fresh every single day. It is absolutely not necessary. When you prepare it, cook enough to last three or four days. This way you will only need to prepare your breakfast porridge two times a week. Store your leftover porridge in your normal leftover containers. You can store it in the refrigerator. Do not use the microwave to reheat your porridge. Simply put the amount of cooked porridge you are going to consume for breakfast in a saucepan or cooking pot and add a little water. Heat over a gentle flame. It only takes a few minutes to heat up your leftover porridge each morning.

Section 2 - Getting Started

🌰 What About Lunch and Dinner?

During Phase One, which will be at least for the duration of your colon cleanse (and then for as many days after that as are needed until your current symptoms are completely gone), you should eat a simple whole foods diet of mostly soups, cooked whole grains and steamed vegetables per the guidelines already provided. This is the only diet that I have found to be completely reliable 100% of the time. Trust me when I tell you that I have seen, heard, and tried every other combination of foods and beverages, sprouts and juices, shakes and smoothies, and there is no other combination that is more reliable than soups, cooked whole grains and steamed vegetables. No coffee, tea, soda, fruit juice, wine, beer, gin, scotch, whiskey. No meat, fish, fruit, beans, cheese, seeds, nuts, flour products and no processed foods of any kind. *This is not forever.* This is only until your symptoms are gone. Once you are symptom-free, you can slowly start adding things back into your diet again. But when you do this, you need to pay very close attention and only add one thing back in at a time to see what effect it has on your digestive system.

There is one other recipe that I have found to be completely compatible with all the other steps and phases of the *Intestinal Regeneration Program*. It is a recipe for miso soup (mee-sew). Miso is a staple of the Japanese diet. It makes all vegetable-based soups into a soothing digestive tonic. It is optional but highly recommended. You can have a small bowl or two before each meal, even breakfast. You can do this during the entire Phase One of your *Intestinal Regeneration Program*. But never eat to fullness. Always leave a little room in your stomach. Get to know this feeling of having eaten enough but not to fullness. Do not overeat. Here is a very basic recipe for miso soup. Feel free to use other vegetables than those listed once you have established this recipe first. Feel free to use the miso soup recipe as part of your breakfast during Phase One if you wish. *When you have miso soup, always consume it first.*

🌰 Basic Miso Soup

Miso is a rich fermented paste made from whole yellow soybeans or occasionally black soybeans, chickpeas or aduki beans alone, or in combination with grains such as barley, brown rice, millet and others. The whole beans and grains are combined with sea salt and natural koji, an enzyme-rich grain that starts the fermentation process. Used in Asia for thousands of years, miso is an excellent aid in the production of healthy intestinal flora. It is rich in microorganisms (probiotics and probiotic conducive materials called prebiotics) and enzymes that strengthen the digestive enzymes and aid in the absorption and assimilation of nutrients in our foods. It also helps in the discharge of toxins from the body by making the elimination of waste more efficient. It is high in protein, calcium, vitamin B, iron, and other nutrients making it an essential food in every healthy whole foods diet.

Basic Miso Soup (approximately four servings)

5 to 6 cups of purified water (don't use tap water)

Some wakame or kombu seaweed (seaweeds are really sea vegetables)

A two inch by two inch square of dried seaweed
per pot of soup is fine

1 large onion, sliced

1 large or two small carrots sliced

1 stalk of celery sliced

3 teaspoons of barley miso (sometimes called Mugi Miso),
organic only

(Miso brands: Westbrae, Eden, Mitoku, South River, Miso Master)

Lightly wash then soak a two inch by two inch strip of dried wakame or kombu until soft. Cut in thin strips and place in cooking water in soup pot. Place sliced onions, carrots and celery in soup pot and bring to boil. Immediately reduce flame to low, cover, and let simmer until onions and carrots are soft. Place three teaspoons of miso in a small bowl (or suribachi if you have one), add some soup broth and puree with a spoon, fork, or pestle until dissolved and creamy. Add this to the rest of the soup and vegetable broth and gently stir. Let simmer for two minutes and then serve. Garnish with fresh cut scallions, flame roasted dulse or nori, or fresh cut parsley. Mmmmm…good.

If and when you reheat your miso soup for the next meal or the next day, make sure that you heat it up slowly and that you do not let the soup bubble or boil. When using miso soup for therapeutic purposes, never overheat and never bring to a boil or this will destroy the beneficial bacteria and enzymes. Miso soup is excellent first thing in the morning and before any meal.

Leftover miso soup can be refrigerated and used for up to three days, after that it should be discarded and a fresh batch made. Try to make only enough for two or three days at a time. The miso package or container can be stored in the refrigerator. Keep sealed. Instant miso products will not be as effective. Please use organic quality miso paste.

Section 2 - Getting Started

🌰 Tamari Tea: Quick Remedy for Gas and Bloating

If you are currently experiencing any abdominal gas or bloating, and/or if you begin to experience any as you start implementing the suggestions in Phase One, there is one very simple remedy that works like a charm to stop abdominal gas within minutes most of the time. It's called Tamari Tea (ta-ma-ree; accent over the ma). Tamari is Japanese soy sauce. Put one half teaspoon of Tamari in a small glass or cup of warm purified water. Stir it up and drink it down. This tea has a very alkalinizing effect and usually works within minutes. If you are still bothered by gas after 15 minutes, try another half teaspoon of tamari in warm water. Then wait at least 30 minutes before trying another cup. This remedy works wherever the gas is located.

What About Other Beverages and Snacks?

Do not drink any other beverages until all your symptoms are gone. Just drink the water from the watercure recipe (plus miso soup and tamari tea as needed). No snacks until all your symptoms are gone. You can snack on soups, porridge and steamed vegetables, (and many people can add organic quality animal protein like chicken and fish). Once you are symptom-free, you can slowly start adding things back into your diet again (some things that is, not all things). When you do this you need to pay very close attention to what you are doing and only add one thing back in at a time to see what effect it has on your digestive system. You can read about my ideas for gradually *Expanding Your Menu Selections in Phase Two* of your program on page 228.

Please Read This Paragraph Before Moving On (Or Giving Up!)

One of the primary difficulties in writing a book that seeks to reflect all the suggestions I make to my clients during their *Intestinal Regeneration Program* is this: everyone is slightly different in their past experiences with whole foods and healing diets in general. What's also true and very important is that everyone's intestinal condition is slightly different. Some people are very sick, meaning their digestive system is very weak and very poorly functioning. These people absolutely need to follow my suggestions as I have been describing them right up to this point. Some people are mildly symptomatic, but right underneath their symptoms their digestive system is actually functioning pretty well. This means that they can be less restrictive in their Phase One food choices. This means that breakfast should be as I have described it for Phase One, but lunch and dinner can be much closer to what they/you are used to. This is an enormous relief to many clients and can make a huge difference in their/your willingness and ability to fully integrate all the rest of my suggestions effectively. What if you are uncertain where you fit in? If you are uncertain choose the stricter dietary path. Read the next section very carefully to get a lot more insight about what you can do to make your program as successful as possible. The next section talks about *the habits of functional nutrition* and addresses the critical issues of when, where, how and why we eat... not just *what* we eat.

Section 2 - Getting Started

🌰 *The Habits of Functional Nutrition*

It's not just *what* you eat, but *how, when, where,* and *why* you eat that makes all the difference in the world! Imagine that.

In the early years of my nutrition counseling career, I was consistently surprised with the number of clients who would tell me something like the following: "I don't know why I am not getting better. I do all the right things. I eat organic whole foods, I don't eat any junk food, I don't drink alcohol, I don't smoke, I exercise a lot, I do yoga, I meditate. What am I missing?" And I would think to myself: "Where is Sherlock Holmes when you need him?" I would answer in the only way I knew how. I would tell them that it didn't make sense to me either. It didn't make sense that they were actually doing all the "right things" and not getting better. Then I would ask them some questions about their diet and lifestyle. Questions designed to elicit their *relationship* to their diet and lifestyle.

Most of us grew up around the cliché, "You are what you eat." And there is definitely a lot of truth to this statement. However, the more I learned about the digestive system, the more I became convinced of a more expanded version of this truism: "We are what we digest, absorb, and assimilate." You could eat the best quality food in the world, prepared with love by the very best organic whole foods chef in the world. All the food could be in perfect balance and proportion, but if you ate too much, or ate too fast, or ate standing up, or ate too late at night, you could end up creating a nightmare of indigestion and all the adverse symptoms related to indigestion. It was very clear to me early on that *how we eat* was as important, and many times, *more important* than *what* we eat.

So, I would ask my clients a few simple questions: Do you chew your food thoroughly? Do you always sit down when you eat? Do you overeat? Do you eat too fast? To which, more often than not, people would answer yes, yes, no, and no, because they knew that these were the correct and preferred answers. I became increasingly suspicious of the stories I was being told by my clients. I wanted to believe they were telling me the truth, but it was becoming abundantly clear that *something* was being lost in the translation between their *perception* of their own reality related to eating, and the real thing.

I call this something an *integrity gap*. An integrity gap happens when you know you should do something but you don't do it. An integrity gap happens when you know you shouldn't do something, but you do it anyway. Some people can easily admit to their integrity gaps but do not perceive the negative influence they exert. Some people are in complete denial about their integrity gaps. They actually know what they are doing, or not doing, but they just won't admit it and make the necessary corrections. And some people are just totally clueless and unconscious of many of the habits they employ and how they affect the digestion, absorption, and assimilation of their foods and beverages.

Helping someone address, correct and ultimately transform their integrity gaps into useful complementary habits are the keys to an effective counseling relationship. It's easy to say, but not always easy to accomplish. For some strange reason, many people seem to resist the transformation of their health and life. Understanding this point is the key to your effectiveness during this program and more importantly for the rest of your life. Your effectiveness is the result of your becoming more proactive in your own self-care.

When I was a new student of natural healing in the mid to late 1970s, I was always conducting "experiments" with everything I was learning about. I felt a powerful need to *prove things* to myself. To find out for sure what worked and what didn't work. To find out for sure, what were the most reliable foods, the most reliable recipes, the most reliable remedies, and the most reliable habits. I would often conduct *experiments* focused on one thing; like chewing each mouthful 100 times. I would do this for seven days, or fourteen days, or twenty-one days. No one had to encourage me to do these things. I was completely self-motivated. I wanted to discover the truth about the real impact of these habits on my digestive system and on my overall health and energy.

When I started counseling others, it did not occur to me to demand that my clients conduct similar experiments on themselves. I think I just assumed that people would do these things on their own, as I had done. And if not, then I would conclude that they just weren't serious enough about getting well. But this was a very unhelpful conclusion on my part. In fact it was a complete lose-lose situation. My client lost out because they simply did not get well. And I lost out, because I did not experience the joy that comes from successfully coaching someone to a condition of better health.

One day something happened to change all that forever. I had been working with a woman in her early fifties, who complained of having indigestion and chronic fatigue. I'll call her Cindy. Cindy was one of those puzzling, well-educated clients I was referring to earlier. She knew everything about nutrition and health. She read all the books. She tried all the diets, all the meditation techniques and all the bodywork therapies. She claimed that nothing had worked. Who was I to doubt her? I believed her. Her case baffled me for months. One lazy Spring afternoon, I got out of work early and drove into town to do a little shopping. I was stopped at a red light, and gazed out the open passenger side window as another car pulled up along side me. It was Cindy. My impulse was to call out to her and say hello, but something stopped me. I kept my mouth shut and just sat and stared at her. I stared because I couldn't believe my eyes. Cindy was sitting in the driver's seat of her car, eating her lunch. I don't know exactly what it was, but it was healthy and wholesome for sure. It was some kind of sandwich. There was big bread involved, with sprouts dangling from the sides. The light changed, and Cindy drove off into the sunset.

As Cindy drove off into the sunset, my mind was buzzing with a thousand realizations! Ok, it was really only one realization, but it felt like a thousand. My realization was this: *What* we eat is not what matters most. What matters most is *how* we eat; and *when* and *where* and *why* we eat. In order for the digestive system to work properly, from start to finish, it has to be relaxed. In order for the digestive system to be relaxed, the person has to be relaxed. In order for the person to relax, he or she must consciously dis-engage from any stressful activity before consuming any food or beverage. I knew this was true from my own personal experience. I knew this was true for all the people I had worked with in the past. I just didn't know how to apply this knowledge more effectively in my current counseling sessions. That all changed the next time I met with Cindy.

Let me make a long story short. The next time I saw Cindy, I gave her an elaborate song and dance about *how we eat* is more important than *what we eat*, and I could tell that she was getting annoyed and bored.

Section 2 - Getting Started

"I know all this!" She insisted. Finally, I was ready to lower the boom. "I know you know all this, Cindy. I am simply concerned that you are not practicing what you know." She was miffed. I then asked her if she ever ate when she was driving her car. She answered immediately: "Never." She said never because she knew this was the correct answer. I then explained to Cindy, that I had caught her red-handed driving her car and eating her lunch the previous Friday afternoon. After we both exchanged glances of mutual embarrassment, and perhaps a little guilt and shame, my face broke out into a huge smile and we both started laughing.

As you have probably already guessed, eating food while driving her car turned out to be the *most insulting habit* in Cindy's diet and lifestyle. Before she left my office that afternoon, I made her promise not to eat anything while driving her car, for *at least* the next 7 days. In fact I made her sign a piece of paper that said: "I will not eat while driving my car for the next seven days." We both signed it. One week later she sat in my office, smiling. "I never would have imagined that one simple, quirky lifestyle habit could have such a powerful effect on my digestion and health. I feel the best I have in years! No more indigestion and no more chronic fatigue. Thank you very much."

This was the first of many similar experiences that were to unfold in the next few years of my nutrition counseling career. Let me summarize a few of my other favorites.

A young woman in her early thirties wanted to get pregnant. I'll call her Beth. She and her husband were happily married and looking forward to starting a family. Beth was about thirty pounds overweight and wanted to lose the weight before getting pregnant. I looked at her diet and could not find any major problems. *What* she was eating seemed fine and *how much* she was eating was also not a problem. In fact I was amazed at how little she ate. Where was all this weight coming from? By this time in my counseling career I had developed a short list of important habits that I would rely upon in these types of situations. I referred to my list as: *the seven habits of highly effective eaters* (with kudos to Stephen Covey).

1. Always say grace at mealtimes (before, during, and after).
2. Always sit down when you eat.
3. Always chew each mouthful completely.
4. Avoid eating or drinking anything too cold.
5. Avoid eating late at night.
6. Avoid processed foods and junk foods and junk beverages.

7. Select the highest quality organic whole foods.

I went down the list as I always did back then, one item at a time, with a brief explanation for each, looking for a *thumbs up* or *thumbs down* from my client. When I got to number four, there was a big thumbs down. Beth started to explain to me about her habit of drinking ice-water. I was amazed. She had a big 24 ounce plastic mug filled with ice in her freezer at all times. Her jug of cold drinking water was always in the refrigerator. She drank ice-water all day long. I knew this was insulting to her digestive system. I did not know it was a contributing factor in her inability to lose weight. I advised her to experiment for a few weeks and only drink room temperature water. In the first 14 days, she lost 15 pounds! After Beth's experience, I knew I was on to something important.

What I learned from Beth's experience was that no habits related to digestion are neutral. I learned that all habits are either complementary and helpful, or they are insulting and harmful in some very specific and measurable ways. I learned that when the digestive system is complemented and functioning normally, it will effectively transform food into nutrients, and then turn the nutrients into useable energy. I learned that when the digestive system is insulted and stressed it becomes inefficient. And one of the adverse effects of digestive inefficiency will be to convert otherwise good food into fat and store it away. And no matter how hard you try to lose that weight, you won't be able to. That is, until you correctly identify the insulting habit and transform it into a complementary habit.

Imagine that.

Then there was David. David called me one night in the middle of the worst sinus congestion he had ever had, and I had ever heard. He was completely stuffed up and very uncomfortable. He was forced to breathe through his mouth. He didn't have any other symptoms, so it was easy to rule out anything too serious, like a viral or bacterial infection. He said he felt fine, he just didn't understand where all the congestion was coming from. David was another one of those well-educated, eco-friendly, holistic-oriented clients, like Cindy. He was a vegetarian by choice. He meditated and did yoga. He was an experienced whole foods cook. All the normal questions about *what* he was eating and *how much* he was eating checked out fine. The causative insult was going to be found somewhere else in his diet and lifestyle. I went down my list of seven habits. David announced that he had just started a new job and during the last three weeks, he was getting home much later than usual and not sitting down for dinner until 9 pm, unlike his normal 6 pm. Aha. I simply suggested that for the next seven days, David not eat anything past 4 pm. He said he would do it. Four days later, he called me on the phone and sounded very different! All the congestion had cleared up completely. This was another big lesson.

It didn't take me long to realize that everyone had at least one or two (or more) of these kinds of *insulting habits* working against them, actively preventing them from getting well. Every day these same habits would reveal themselves in my counseling sessions and more often than not, turn out to be the critical piece of information that allowed everything else to work, and opened the door to the successful self-healing of my clients.

It didn't take me long to realize that learning the difference between the complementary and insulting habits (and influences) in our diet and lifestyle represents one of the most important things we will ever learn. Practicing the complementary habits and avoiding the insulting habits *is the difference* between healing ourselves and staying sick.

Imagine that.

🌰 Complementary or Insulting?

What are the habits of naturally healthy people according to the principles of functional nutrition?

This step of your *Intestinal Regeneration Program* is the most important step of all. If you fail to identify your most insulting habits (and then avoid them) you may not experience the success you desire and deserve. If you fail to avoid your most insulting habits during the Phase One recovery period, you may not recover your normal intestinal functions. However, if you take this step seriously and practice the complementary habits while avoiding the insulting ones, you will be astonished at how rapidly your intestinal regeneration will proceed. This step, in my opinion, is what makes my program different and more effective than any other. This step integrates your bio-chemical individuality with all your dietary and lifestyle idiosyncrasies. This step customizes and personalizes your program making it unique and special. Other books and programs and practitioners give *lip service* to some of these habits but generally overlook their *primary* significance. These habits aren't just important: *they are transformational.* In my experience all the habits listed below provide the keys to your self-healing journey. Separate the complementary habits from the insulting ones, practice the complementary habits and minimize or avoid the insulting ones and you will dramatically increase your recovery time. Please read this next section very carefully. Please read this next section as if your entire digestive system health depended on it. It does.

We are what we repeatedly do.
Excellence then, is not an act, but a habit.
Aristotle

Practice These
Complementary Habits Consistently!

- Think before you eat or drink anything always: "What nourishes me best?"
- Select the highest quality foods and beverages always. Organic quality is best.
- Learn how and why to select and prepare your foods and beverages according to the principles of balance and harmony in nature. Find the best whole foods cooking instructors in your area and take some classes.
- Always say *Grace* with any meal or snack. Grace is the pause that nourishes best. If you believe in God, saying *Grace* is probably a no brainer, a given. Or it could be one of those major *integrity gaps* that needs your attention. But whether or not you believe in God, or whether or not you belong to any religion, saying *Grace* is still important and makes good common sense. Where did this food come from that I am about to consume? Where is it going? Why? You don't have to call this habit *Grace*. You can call it anything you want. Just make sure you stop before you begin to consume any meal, beverage, or snack. Make sure you ask these three questions: Where did this (food, beverage, snack, supplement, etc) come from? Where is it going? Why? If you do this consistently, this habit will change your life.
- Create an atmosphere of peace and quiet, relaxation and calmness around mealtimes. Light a candle. Put on some quiet music. Turn off the TV. Turn off the radio news. Shut off the phone. Don't answer the phone during mealtimes. Don't eat when you are angry, upset, stressed-out or tired. First you must relax. Go for a walk,

clear you head, breathe. Don't let mealtime be invaded by other time. Mealtimes are special. Mealtimes are sacred.

- Learn to breathe from your belly. This habit will not only help you relax, it will help you to digest everything better.
- Always sit down when you eat. Eating standing up or on the run (or in the car) is one of the best and fastest ways I know to create indigestion.
- Enjoy regular mealtimes. Create balance in your day. Seek harmony in your daily activities. Look to the rhythms in nature and discover how they relate to your life.
- Approach each meal with an attitude of gratitude. How lucky am I to have such abundance and variety in my meal options? How lucky am I to have farmers who know how to grow such wonderful food? How lucky am I to have a fully functioning digestive system that knows exactly what to do with all this wonderful food! This is a form of, or an extension of *grace* with meals.
- Take your Essentials supplements before meals.
- Don't dine without your supplemental digestive enzymes.
- Eat one mouthful at a time. Put less food on your fork or spoon. Eat less, chew more. Put down your fork, spoon, knife, or chopsticks between mouthfuls. Chew each mouthful until your food becomes liquid in your mouth. Slow down. Eat less, chew more. This habit is so extremely important I am going to repeat it.
- Chew each mouthful of food completely. Eat one mouthful at a time. Put your fork down between mouthfuls. Slow down. Drink your solids and chew your liquids. There may be no greater dietary *integrity gap* than this one. (We all know that chewing is important but we rarely do it!) The good news is this: Consistent proper chewing of every mouthful of food you consume produces extraordinary health benefits that you simply cannot imagine possible until you experience them yourself directly. Experiment, and experience the benefits! Chew, chew, chew!
- Your stomach can expand quite a bit to accommodate your overeating of large quantities of food. It doesn't want to do this. This should be the exception not the rule. Unfortunately it is a very common practice these days. Traditional peoples taught themselves the habit of knowing when to stop eating, before fullness. Your normal stomach is about the size of your clenched fist. Right. Not very big. You need to learn to eat slowly and only until your stomach is about 75–80% full. Learning the art of when

to stop eating is as important as learning the art of when to start eating. This habit will teach you humility, kindness and generosity.

- Practice the habit of proper daily hydration according to the watercure recipe described earlier in this section.
- Exercise. Exercise moderately and frequently. Walking every day for 20 to 30 minutes may be all that most people require. It's a start, and a very good one at that. Exercise increases oxygen levels in our blood and throughout the cells of our entire body. Oxygen is another one of those most fundamental internal regulators and biomodulators. Almost every function in the human body requires water and oxygen.
- Moderate exercise is also the very best way to circulate our lymphatic fluid, bringing necessary nutrients to cells and removing undesirable toxic waste matter away from cells. Our blood supply has a pump called the heart, but we have twice the amount of lymph fluid in our body and the only pump is moderate daily exercise.
- Learn how to give yourself a therapeutic abdominal massage.
- Get enough sleep at night and rest during the day if necessary. If you need a nap, take one. Napping is extremely therapeutic especially if you are healing. Most people require eight hours of sleep at night and the most important hours of sleep are those before midnight. If you stay up too late you will not get better. Go to bed earlier for a week and see what a difference it makes. Pay attention to the natural rhythms of the rising and setting of the sun and moon. Go to sleep after sunset. Try to get up an hour before sunrise. See what a difference this habit makes.
- Conduct an effective 7-14 day colon cleanse at least once every year and preferably once every season, that is, after completing the colon cleanse from Phase One.
- Start and keep a daily journal of self-discovery. This journal can chronicle your ongoing process of distinguishing complementary habits from insulting ones. This journal can chronicle the people, places, and things that nourish you best.

Section 2 - Getting Started

🌰 Avoid These Insulting Habits as Much as Possible!

- Avoid wearing tight pants. Don't laugh. It is absolutely amazing to me how many people fail to understand and observe this most basic, most sensible of habits. You may think this is silly and obvious, but you would be amazed how many people make how they look more important than how they feel. Any restriction of your abdomen, especially after a meal is going to cause problems. (Remember Jessica's story?) Your belly must remain relaxed and not constricted at all times if you are going to heal yourself from any digestive problem. Wear loose fitting undergarments and loose fitting pants or skirts. Don't wear your belt too tight. You will be rewarded greatly for paying attention to this very important detail.
- Avoid eating anything too late in the day. Remember the story of the king, the prince and the pauper. Eat like a king at breakfast, a prince at lunch, and a pauper at dinner! How late is too late? It varies from person to person and condition to condition. Any time after sunset is risky. Simply keep in mind that the digestive system works best during the daylight hours. When you experiment with this habit you will see just how powerful it is. For so many people, the habit of eating late at night is their major insult, and changing this habit is the key to their success.
- Avoid eating or drinking anything too cold. What's too cold? Again it varies from person to person and condition to condition. Simply keep in mind that the entire digestive system is functioning at 98.6 degrees (and warmer) and is moist and humid like a tropical rainforest. No ice water, ice cream, frozen yogurt, iced drinks. Many symptoms associated with indigestion have their "root cause" right here. When your digestive health is really poor, this habit is

absolutely critical to your improvement. Once you are well again, you will have to experiment and see how things affect you. Do this with all the habits. Experiment.

- Avoid excess meat and dairy consumption. Choose quality. Find the balance.
- Avoid alcohol, cigarettes, caffeine. Not for the rest of your life. Just today. Just one day at a time.
- Avoid processed and synthetic foods and beverages. Read labels. Avoid junk food.
- Avoid all toxins in our food, air, water, clothing, and household cleaning products, synthetic carpets and furniture, suspect gardening products, and building supplies.
- Avoid excess consumption of fruit juice from concentrates especially with children. Concentrated juices may concentrate nutrients but they concentrate sugars too.
- Avoid all carbonated beverages. $CO2$ (carbon dioxide) is a toxic by-product of normal human metabolic activity. We breathe in oxygen and we breathe out carbon dioxide. This is one of those insane modern inventions that represent *giant leaps backwards* when it comes to the combination of nutrition and technology. The body works incredibly hard to get rid of carbon dioxide from our blood. Why on earth would we want to put carbon dioxide back into our body?
- Avoid Aspartame and other synthetic and artificial sweeteners.
- Avoid artificial colors, additives, preservatives, fortifiers, fillers. We must consume real foods, whole foods, not fake foods.
- Avoid the use of artificial and synthetic placeware, cookware, and utensils. Use wood, ceramic, glass, cast iron, stainless steel.
- Avoid the use of artificial cooking techniques in general and microwave cooking in particular.
- Avoid the habit of consuming a mono diet as in monotonous. Variety is an important nutritional requirement, perhaps as important as any other. Too many people eat the same things day after day, breakfast, lunch and dinner; month after month, winter, spring, summer, and fall; year after year, through childhood, adolescence, maturity, and old age. Don't do this to yourself! The more dynamic and flexible your food choices are the greater the variety of beneficial bacteria and vital foods enzymes will be. Variety complements the proper functioning of your digestive system. Variety is the spice of life! Obviously, during Phase One

of your *Intestinal Regeneration Program* your menu selections will be purposefully limited. So this habit is really an invitation to those who successfully complete Phase One and Phase Two.
- Review the habits checklist regularly on pages 259-262.

There is substantial and reliable documentation to support each of the habits outlined above (see the bibliography). However, nothing is more important and ultimately nothing is more convincing than the actual *experiments* you conduct yourself *on yourself* to determine the relevance of any of these habits. If you are not willing to carry out experiments with your diet and your habits, as explained below, you will only see limited improvement or none at all. You must conduct reliable experiments to prove to yourself *conclusively* which habits in your diet and lifestyle are complementary and which ones are insulting. Your health depends on these experiments. Please use the following suggestions to guide your experiments.

The Seven Day Experiment

Seven Days is the absolute minimum period of time to conduct a meaningful experiment.
1. Pick a habit that you want to experiment with from the list above.
2. Make an unbreakable commitment to experiment with 100% enthusiasm and integrity. This means that *no matter what* comes up in your life in the form of any distraction whatsoever, you will not break your commitment to your experiment.
3. Let's say you have decided to conduct a chewing experiment. You obviously cannot avoid chewing, so you simply decide to chew more diligently and more completely than ever before. Not just for one or two meals, but for every meal, beverage and snack during the next seven days. You will be amazed at your results. To be effective you must count your chews. Don't swallow until each mouthful has turned to liquid. Eat only one mouthful at a time. Put your fork down between mouthfuls. In other words, *eat with total awareness, sensitivity, and consciousness!*
4. If you need to, write down your commitment to yourself and sign it. Put it on the wall of your bedroom or office or the bathroom mirror. Have your wife sign it, or your husband. If you need to, get it witnessed and notarized. Do whatever you need to do to make, and then keep, your unbreakable seven day commitment to yourself.
5. Don't *try* to do this seven day experiment. Just do it! Get serious. Be real. Follow through. I can't tell you how many clients tell me: "Oh, I just couldn't do it. This came up and that came up and blah, blah, blah." I say nonsense. I say; "balderdash." Excuses are

just excuses. Personal healing requires personal power, the power to choose and decide what nourishes us best and what doesn't. No one ever healed themselves by not following through. No one ever healed themselves by just trying. No one ever grew a magnificent garden without weeding and composting. Insulting habits are weeds. Complementary habits are compost. If you are not willing to identify the weeds in your life and pull them out by the roots, they will eventually take over your garden. You cannot let the weeds in your life dictate what your garden is going to look and feel like. You must cultivate the habits that nourish you best. Become a master gardener. Separate the weeds from the things you most want to grow. You will be amazed at how successful you can become at this.

I hear and I forget. I do and I understand.
Chinese proverb

Section 2 - Getting Started

The Power of Choice:
Your Key To a Successful Phase One

It is simply a statement of fact and a matter of principle to say that you are in your current condition because of the choices you have made up until the present time. No guilt, no blame, no shoulda, coulda, woulda. You are where you are and you are experiencing what you are currently experiencing. It is what it is. You cannot change the past. Imagine that.

It is also a statement of fact and a matter of principle to say that if your future is going to be different than your past, and better and healthier than your past, you are going to have to make different and better choices. You are going to have to make different and better choices about who you are and why you are here. You are going to have to make different and better choices about what your body is and how it works and what it needs. You are going to have to make different and better choices about what nourishes you best. I believe sincerely that you can do this. I have absolutely no doubt in my mind that you can do this!

> *I believe sincerely that every person has consummate genius within them. Self-awareness of this fact allows for greatness or holds people down to mediocrity. I believe that mediocrity is self-inflicted and that genius is self-bestowed. The key is desire!*
> Walter Russell

Desire, choice, personal power, commitment, decisiveness, imagination, resourcefulness, flexibility. You will need all of these things and many more if you are going to successfully heal yourself of your digestive system problems. It has taken me forty years (since 1973) to discover the effectiveness of all the information, suggestions and habits in the first two sections of this book. As the old saying goes: "You can lead a horse to water, but you can't make him drink." I am confident that you can heal yourself using the guidelines and suggestions in this book. And of course, there is more supportive information in Section Three. Ultimately, your success is going to be determined by the choices you make from this moment forward. Nothing is ever going to change this most basic fact of our existence: Success in life is determined by the choices we make about everything, moment to moment to moment.

At one of the lowest moments in the early days of my healing journey, I had a remarkable experience. This experience taught me how quickly things can change when the mind finally lets go of old habits and allows the insight of a new idea to penetrate, illuminate and transform one's consciousness and one's entire being. This experience taught me that these things can happen at any time; especially in a moment and under circumstances when you might least expect such kinds of things to happen.

Even if you are on the right track, if you just sit there,
you'll get run over!
Will Rogers

The Power of Our Core Beliefs

It was 1978. I was twenty-three years old. I was working a part-time job, trying to save up some money so I could leave home and take the next step in my healing journey. I was working on an assembly line stuffing annual stock reports from AT&T into 50 pound mail bags. We were not supposed to eat any food on the assembly line. Managers were constantly walking around making sure everything was being done according to the rules. I had just returned from a break and was taking the last few bites of an apple. I turned the corner of the hallway and saw one of the managers coming towards me. Without thinking I popped the rest of the apple into my mouth and pretended I wasn't eating anything. I walked by the manager. He didn't notice anything peculiar, but I did.

I never ate the core of the apple. So this was a new experience for me. I started chewing, biting down into the apple pits. My entire life, right up until that moment, I had never made the distinction between apple *pits* and apple *seeds*. I learned about apple pits, peach pits, apricot pits and that I was not supposed to eat them. But the point here is this: I never once considered the fact that an apple pit is the same thing as an apple seed. Pits were things you discarded. Pits were things you avoided. Pits were not good. Pits were worthless. Pits had no redeeming value whatsoever. Imagine that.

It didn't matter whether these things were true or not. These were habits in my own personal thinking based upon some old core beliefs. Where these beliefs came from I did not know; from my family most likely, maybe from my culture. It didn't matter. What mattered was that my beliefs about pits completely determined my imagination about pits. And what I was used to imagining about pits determined my behavior about pits.

Walking down the hall that day, chewing on a mouthful of apple pits I realized that I had never examined my core beliefs about pits before. I just accepted the images, thoughts and feelings I had about pits, as if they were true. It had simply never occurred to me to re-examine my core beliefs about pits before that moment. Imagine that.

Imagination is more important than knowledge.
Albert Einstein

Why am I telling you this story? I have shared with you earlier in the book that one of the biggest health challenges in my life was and had been my battles with anxiety and depression. The image I had in my mind about depression was that depression was a deep dark pit: like the pit in Edgar Allan Poe's story, *The Pit and the Pendulum;* like that final scene in the 1940s movie, *The Snake Pit.* Depression was a pit and the only way out was up. Every day I experienced depression, I imagined myself clawing my way up the sides of a big, black, slimy, stinking pit. The pit of depression I was in was a loathsome, hateful, fearful place. There wasn't anything positive or helpful about it. The pit of depression I was in was a living hell. The only thing I wanted to do with the pit was to get out of it and go as far away from it as possible and never go back. Pits sucked. That was my basic core belief about pits. Pits sucked the life from people. Pits were bad.

No matter how much effort I exerted in trying to get out of my pit of depression, I never got out. The more effort I exerted the more exhausted I became. The more exhausted I became, the more hopeless I became. As a result, I started to believe that I might never get out. This was the scariest thought of all. This kind of growing inclination bordering on conviction was putting me deeper into hell and further and further away from any effective help. Beliefs determine behavior. My unexamined beliefs about the pits of depression were not helping me at all. In truth, my core beliefs about depression pits and the images they conjured in my mind were sucking the life-energy out of me.

So there I was, biting down and gnashing the pits of my apple core, when for the very first time in my life, I realized that an *apple pit* was actually an *apple seed...* a seed! Suddenly my dark and horror-filled imagination and consciousness was bursting with the light from a thousand stars. I calmly walked away from the assembly line and went straight to the men's room. I needed a little rest from all my sudden internal excitement. I took out my little notebook and pen from the back pocket of my jeans and wrote down the following words:

> I dove into an empty pit!
> Big, black, abysmal.
> Half-way in
> I discovered I was half-way out,
> And the empty pit I thought I was dying in
> Became a seed
> Through which I was giving birth
> To my new self!

Prior to that moment I had never even remotely considered that there might be another way of looking at the pit of my deep dark depression. For the first time in my life I was choosing to consider that the deep dark pit of my depression might also be serving as some kind of protective cave in which I (or some aspect of my consciousness) had simply been resting and waiting for the appropriate time to re-emerge; like the proverbial bear from hibernation, like the butterfly from its cocoon, like the first green shoots of spring. As a result of this realization, I started feeling really hopeful again for the first time in what had been a very long time without much hope.

If I had been so wrong about my limiting beliefs about the lowly apple pit, how many other wrong beliefs might I also have? I found myself asking this question often in the days following my illuminating apple-pit, apple-seed experience. And how were these other beliefs of mine affecting my behavior? How were my other beliefs affecting my choices and decisions? How were my other beliefs affecting my life and my desire to be healthy and happy and whole again? I started to examine my core beliefs about everything. A funny thing happened as a result of this constant examination of my life and core beliefs. My life and health started to improve dramatically. Imagine that!

The unexamined life is not worth living.
Socrates

You just never know when these kinds of things are going to happen to you. But you have to have the belief that they *might happen* to you or you may not be paying attention when they do.

Beliefs determine our behavior.

This is one of the great insights of all time. If you do not believe that you are going to get well, you may not get well. If you do not believe that you deserve to get well, you may not get well. If you do not believe that you have the capacity to make the right choices for yourself, you may not make the right choices. If you do not believe that your deepest feelings about things matter, you may not *summon up* the desire and the will to change your condition and circumstances.

Beliefs determine our behavior.

You must give yourself permission to choose new beliefs and re-examine old ones. You must determine which beliefs will support your self-healing journey and which ones will not. You must! You must! You must!

You must focus on, activate, and *compost* the beliefs that support you. You must weed out the beliefs that don't support you. Put your shovel in the earth, turn it over, and move on. Keep cultivating the soil of your own life. Keep choosing the habits and beliefs that nourish you best.

To every thing, turn, turn, turn.
There is a season, turn, turn, turn,
And a time for every purpose under heaven.
Pete Seeger

You must remember that one definition of insanity is this: to continue to do the same things over and over again, hoping for a different result. You are at an important crossroads in your healing journey. You must change directions. You must do it now. You must simply discover the things that nourish you best and then consistently do the things that nourish you best.

If not now, when? If not me, then who?
Rabbi Hillel

To successfully change your life you must examine your beliefs. To successfully examine your beliefs you must step outside of your regular routines and seek the counsel of your deepest innermost being. To successfully do this you're going to need some quiet time alone. I suggest you go for a walk in the woods. I suggest you find a path less traveled by and take it. I promise you it will make all the difference in the world.

The Road Not Taken

Two roads diverged in a yellow wood,
And sorry I could not travel both
And be one traveler, long I stood
And looked down one as far as I could
To where it bent in the undergrowth;

Then took the other, as just as fair,
And having perhaps the better claim,
Because it was grassy and wanted wear;
Though as for that, the passing there
Had worn them really about the same,

And both that morning equally lay
In leaves no step had trodden black.
Oh, I kept the first for another day!
Yet knowing how way leads on to way,
I doubted if I should ever come back.

I shall be telling this with a sigh
Somewhere ages and ages hence;
Two roads diverged in a wood, and I
I took the one less traveled by,
And that has made all the difference.

Robert Frost

Section Three
OPTIMIZING RESULTS

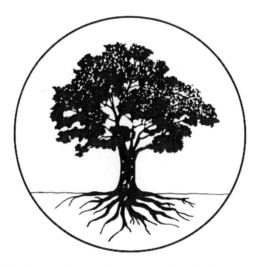

Food is the soil from which the tree of our own life is grown.

🌰 The Purpose of Section Three

The purpose of Section Three is to provide fuller, broader, and deeper information and explanations for the ideas and suggestions discussed in Sections One and Two. In situations where the original information is already comprehensive, I will just provide brief summaries to highlight the most important points. Please take note where some of the articles appearing in Section Three have been written by other health writers.

The Modern Cornucopia

The cornucopia or horn of plenty is the traditional and ancient symbol of the harvest. It is also a symbol of abundance. The healthiest diet is a diet that consists mostly of organic quality whole foods. These would be the foods found in the traditional cornucopia. Too many of our modern food selections are highly processed and packaged foods. These foods by and large are lacking vitality, lacking enzymes, lacking nutrients and more than likely play host to a variety of additives and preservatives. Non-organic foods may contain residues of pesticides and herbicides and other non-nutritious and potentially toxic substances. Common sense leads us to select foods that have been enjoyed for thousands of years and have stood the tests of time and billions of discerning minds and palates. The list below is representative not exhaustive. Most of the foods listed are available in organic versions. Keep in mind that each category of certain foods can have hundreds of varieties. In China there are thousands of varieties of rice for example. And how could we possibly list all the varieties of grapes used in wine-making? Too many to list!

Whole Foods: whole grains like rice, wheat, oats, barley, rye, corn, amaranth, quinoa, millet, buckwheat, wild rice, teff, bulghur; beans and legumes like kidney beans, lentils, split peas, lima beans, navy beans, mung beans, pinto beans, aduki beans, soy beans, black beans, garbanzo beans; vegetables like string beans, asparagus, broccoli, mushrooms, potatoes, tomatoes, eggplant, zucchini, jerusalem artichoke, turnip, beets, brussel sprouts, cabbage, carrots, cauliflower, cucumber, onions, garlic, shallots, leeks, okra, parsnips, green peppers, red peppers, chili peppers, radish, pumpkin, summer squash, spaghetti

Section 3 - Optimizing Results

squash, hubbard squash, buttercup squash, butternut squash, acorn squash, sweet potato, yam, rutabaga, burdock root, ginger root, daikon, snowpeas, avocado, bok choy, chinese cabbage, kale, collard greens, kohlrabi, mustard greens, turnip greens, beet greens, alfalfa sprouts, various bean sprouts, wheat grass, chives, swiss chard, parsley, endive, romaine lettuce, iceberg lettuce, spinach, watercress; sea vegetables like dulse, wakame, kelp, kombu, nori, hijiki, arame; seeds and nuts like almonds, brazil nuts, cashews, chestnuts, coconut, hazelnuts, hickory nuts, filberts, macadamia nuts, peanuts, pecans, pine nuts, pistachios, walnuts, pumpkin seeds, sunflower seeds, sesame seeds, squash seeds; fruits like apples (so many varieties!), apricots, bananas, blackberries, blueberries, boysenberries, cherries, crabapple, dates, cranberries, currants, elderberries, figs, gooseberries, grapefruit, grapes, guava, kiwi, kumquats, lemons, limes, loganberries, loquats, lychee, mango, melons (cantaloupe, casaba, honeydew, watermelon, cranshaw), mulberries, nectarines, oranges, papaya, passion fruit, peaches, pears, persimmons, pineapple, plantain, plum, pomegranate, prune, prickly pear, quince, raisins, raspberries, rhubarb, strawberries, tangerines. Are you eating a variety of all of these foods?

Animal foods: beef, calves liver, chuck roast, corned beef, flank steak, rib roast, ground beef, hamburger meat, porterhouse steak, round steak, short ribs, sirloin steak, t-bone steak, tenderloin, veal cutlet, lamb (various cuts), pork (various cuts), bacon, Canadian bacon, pork feet, pork knuckles, pork chop, spare ribs, ham, sweetbreads, rump roast, rabbit, venison, chicken, duck (breast, back, leg, thigh, wing, liver), goose, pheasant, quail, turkey, fish (abalone, anchovy, bass, bluefish, carp, catfish, caviar, cod, eel, flounder, haddock, halibut, herring, mackerel, perch, pike, pollock, salmon, sardines, shark, smelt, snails, snapper, sole, swordfish, trout, tuna, white-fish), shellfish (clams, conch, crab, crawfish, lobster, oysters, scallops, shrimp), processed meats (bologna, bratworst, frankfurter, Italian sausage, kielbasa, knockwurst, liverwurst, mortadella, pepperoni, pork and beef sausages, Polish sausage, salami, Vienna sausage), goose liver pate, duck liver pate, various other pates, chicken eggs, goose eggs, cow's milk, goat's milk and various cheeses made from these milks (American cheese, bleu, brick, brie, camembert, cheddar, cheshire, colby, cottage cheese, cream cheese, edam, feta, fontina, gouda, gruyere, limburger, Monterrey jack, mozzarella, muenster, neufchatel, parmesan, provolone, ricotta, romano, roquefort, Swiss), other milk and dairy products (butter, buttermilk, eggnog, half and half, heavy cream, ice cream, ice milk, milk [lowfat, skim, and whole], sour cream, whipping cream, yogurt). Let me know if I have missed something.

Processed Foods: Since we rarely consume any entire animal, many of the foods listed in the animal foods category above can also be consider processed foods. When we are seeking quality and vitality in our food selections, the closer the food in question is to the actual harvest date the better. Think of picking an apple from a tree, grapes from the vine, or carrots from the field. As time passes from the point of harvest of any food, animal or vegetable, that food loses vitality, energy, enzymes, and nutrients. Fresh whole foods in season are always the best choices to make. Listed are various types of processed foods by category.

Fats and oil: beef tallow, butter, margarine, vegetable shortening, lard, bacon fat, corn oil, olive oil, peanut oil, safflower oil, sesame oil, soybean oil, sunflower oil, oils from certain herbs that are becoming increasingly popular but are used as nutritional supplements, not for cooking (evening primrose oil and borage oil for example). When choosing a cooking and baking oil it is better to choose organic quality, cold-pressed oils over hydrogenated oils. Nut butters such as peanut butter. Nut butters can be made from any seed or nut. See the whole foods list above.

Salad dressings and sauces: bleu cheese, French, Italian, mayonnaise, Russian, thousand island, various barbecue sauces, Worcestershire sauce, tamari, soy sauce, ketchup, mustard, vinegar (rice vinegar, apple cider vinegar, white vinegar, balsamic vinegar, etc.) Obviously this is a very partial list!

Processed grain products, bakery items, flour products: buckwheat flour, carob, corn flour, wheat gluten, pastry flour from various wheat berries, peanut flour, rice flour, rye flour, barley flour, oat flour, pearled barley, scotch oats, steel cut oats, rolled oats, bulghur, cracked wheat, corn meal, cornstarch, popcorn, tapioca, pasta, spaghetti, macaroni, linguini, fettucini, rigatoni, cornbread, bagels, biscuits, English muffins, pita bread, dinner rolls, wheat bread, rye bread, pumpernickel, hot dog rolls, hamburger rolls, submarine rolls, graham crackers, soda crackers, oyster crackers, saltine crackers, bran muffins, blueberry muffins, corn muffins, whole wheat pancakes, buckwheat pancakes, crepes, pizza crust, pretzels, taco shells, tortilla, waffles, bran flakes, corn flakes, puffed corn, granola, oat flakes, puffed oats, puffed rice, rice crackers, cream of wheat, wheat germ, shredded wheat, puffed wheat, wheat granules, grapenuts, angel food cake, devil's food cake, pound cake, gingerbread cake, sponge cake, white cake, cookies of all kinds, brownies, doughnuts of all kinds, pastries of all kinds, pie crusts of all kinds, etc.

Sweeteners, chocolates, candy bars, hard candy: maple syrup of many grades and varieties, honey (many varieties), corn syrup, molasses, white sugar, brown sugar, raw sugar, cane sugar, confectioners sugar, stevia root, artificial sugars like Nutrasweet and Equal (Aspartame), fruit jams and jellies, chocolates, fudge, chocolate pudding, hard candy of all kinds, chewing gum and bubble gum of all kinds, salt water taffy, etc.

Pickled and fermented foods: pickled vegetables, pickled fruit, pickled eggs, all kinds of pickles, kimchi, sauerkraut, miso, tempeh, tamari, yogurt, kefir, etc.

Soups: vegetable soups of endless variety, black bean soup, beef bouillon, beef noodle, cream of celery, chicken broth, cream of chicken, chicken gumbo, chicken noodle, clam chowder, gazpacho, lentil soup, minestrone, cream of mushroom, onion soup, oyster stew, split pea soup, cream of potato soup, tomato soup, turkey noodle, etc.

Beverages, all kinds: beer of endless variety, wine of endless variety, cordials and liqueurs, gin, vodka, rum, bourbon, whiskey, rye, scotch, club soda, tonic water, ginger ale, cola, endless variety of carbonated beverages, carbonated waters, purified water, coffee of many varieties, teas including herbal teas of endless varieties, fruit juice of all varieties, vegetable juice of all varieties and combinations, dairy milk, soy milk, nut milk, coconut milk, etc. The best beverage for health purposes is purified water with sea salt.

Other things appearing in our food supply: Additives, preservatives, flavor enhancers, stabilizers, thickeners, enrichers, growth hormones, antibiotics, and genetically modified organisms (GMOs) do not appear in organic quality whole foods. These materials, and others not listed here, which are not essential nutrients, appear in conventionally grown foods, processed foods, and junk foods. These materials appear in our food supply even when the manufacturer claims the product to be "natural." The "natural" label is both meaningless and misleading. The only valid distinction for any healthy food is whether it is whole or processed and whether it is certified organic, or not. If not, then you simply take your chances as to how it was grown and processed and whether it is making a healthy contribution to your body or not.

A Word to the Wise: Try to remember that the foods we select and prepare for eating are being eaten for the health of our bodies, minds, and spirits. All the materials and ingredients found in our foods, eventually find their way into our cells, becoming our selves. Reflect wisely before you select, prepare, and consume any food or beverage. Reflect afterwards about how the food, beverage, snack, or meal makes you feel, immediately afterwards and hours later too. Start making the connections between what you eat and how you feel and think and dream. We are not only what we eat, but how, when, where, and why we eat. We are the result of what our digestive system is able to break down, absorb, and assimilate. The micronutrients from our foods and beverages make up the physical structures of our cells, tissues, organs, and systems. Healthy food and complementary habits are a great blessing and the key to happiness and longevity. What are the foods and habits that nourish us best?

Source for food lists: John D. Kirschman with Lavon J.Dunne, *Nutrition Almanac* [New York: McGraw Hill, 1984], 242–281)

Section 3 - Optimizing Results

🌰 The Truth About Whole Grains

As explained briefly on page 149 in Section Two, whole grains are seeds. You can put them in fertile soil, add some water and sunlight and they will sprout And they will do this even after many years in storage. This is one reason why they were prized so highly by ancient and traditional peoples around the world. When archeologists found the pyramids in Egypt in the late nineteenth century, whole grains of wheat and rice were found buried with the pharaohs. These grains were still potent after thousands of years!

Whole grains have been the most important staple food for most human beings on planet earth for at least the last ten thousand years. The archeological records show that the earliest villages and towns started when and where whole grains could be dependably grown and harvested. Civilization and modern culture begin with agriculture. If you pick up any of the major American news or gossip magazines, you will see a proliferation of ads touting the benefits of whole grains; vitamins, minerals, energy, fiber; even lowering cholesterol! However, the products being touted in these ads are not whole grains. They are highly refined and processed food products made from whole grains. So don't be fooled. If your digestive system is weak, suffering, or impaired in any way you need to avoid all forms of processed grain products until you regain your normal digestive function. And then, use processed grain products sparingly. The nutritional value of any processed grain product is negligible, even organic quality processed grain products. Cooked whole grains are always better than processed grains.

Here is a short but reliable list of processed grain products you will want to avoid for a while and possibly forever: every breakfast cereal that comes in a box or a bag including things like granola, muesli, oatmeal, wheat flakes, oat flakes and corn flakes. Did you ever stop to think how these various grain flakes were made? First they mill the grain into flour. Then they reconstitute the flour into a flake. Then they add the vitamins and minerals and usually some preservative or the flakes will wilt quickly. Wheat puffs, rice puffs, corn puffs, and other puffed grains are also to be avoided. Popcorn, if you make it yourself from whole organic corn, can be a great snack, but I would wait until Phase Two to try it. Avoid rice cakes, steel cut oats, rolled oats, and rolled barley. Almost every processed breakfast cereal that is not actually a certified organic whole grain in bulk form is not conducive to digestive system health and could be actively insulting and detrimental to your healing process.

It is a travesty that the major cereal manufacturers can get away with promoting their products as whole grains when they are in fact processed grains. There is no comparable value nutritionally at all. It's apples and oranges. It's seeds vs dust. Once you take that seed of a whole grain and grind it into flour, or press it into a flake, or blow it into a puff you no longer have a whole grain. You have a highly refined and processed food product made from whole grains. It is best to avoid all processed grain products until you have fully restored normal functioning to your digestive system. This means avoiding things like, bread, cereal, muffins, cake, pies, cookies, donuts, pasta, noodles, and macaroni. This change does not usually mean forever; just until your digestive system normalizes. Simply keep in mind that nutritionally speaking, cooked whole grains are always going to be the superior foods and almost always complementary if prepared correctly and consumed correctly while processed grains are always going to be inferior and insulting to one degree or another. Imagine that.

Toxicology and Human Health

What are the major hazards we face as human beings?

- *Cultural hazards* such as unsafe working conditions, smoking, poor diet, drugs, drinking, driving, criminal assault, unsafe sex and poverty.
- *Chemical hazards* from harmful chemicals in the air, water, and food.
- *Physical hazards* such as noise, fire, tornadoes, hurricanes, earthquakes, volcanic eruptions, floods, droughts and ionizing radiation.
- *Biological hazards* from pathogens (bacteria, viruses and parasites), pollen and other allergens and insects and animals such as bees and poisonous snakes.

(In this brief excerpt the focus is on chemical hazards. This article has been taken from a textbook called, *Living in the Environment*. More details about the book at the end of the article.)

What are toxic and hazardous chemicals?

Toxic chemicals are generally defined as substances that are fatal to over 50% of test animals at given concentrations. Hazardous chemicals cause harm in at least four ways:

1. By being flammable or explosive
2. By being irritating or damaging to the skin or lungs (gasoline)
3. By interfering with or preventing oxygen uptake and distribution, such as in the case of asphyxiants like carbon monoxide and hydrogen sulfide
4. By inducing allergic reactions of the immune system, as in anaphylactic shock, which can be caused by bee stings, snake bites, and allergic reactions to peanuts and strawberries and other foods by certain people.

According to the World Health Organization, environmental and lifestyle factors play a key role in causing or promoting up to 80% of all cancers. Major sources of carcinogens are cigarette smoke (30-40% of cancers), diet (20-30%), occupational exposure (5-15%) and environmental pollutants (1-10%). About 10-20% of cancers are believed to be caused by inherited genetic factors (5%) or by certain viruses. (These statistics are changing as we learn more about the ill-effects of various environmental pollutants.)

Typically, 10 to 40 years may elapse between the initial exposure to a carcinogen and the appearance of detectable symptoms. Partly because of this time lag, many healthy teenagers (and young adults) have trouble believing that their smoking, drinking, eating, and other lifestyle habits today, could lead to some form of cancer later on.

Synthetic chemicals which threaten the Nervous System: (a few examples)

- Chlorinated hydrocarbons like DDT, PCBs, dioxins
- Organophosphate pesticides
- Formaldehyde
- Various compounds of arsenic, mercury, lead, and cadmium
- Widely used industrial solvents such as TCE (trichloroethylene), toluene, and xylene

In 1995 researchers in the Netherlands found a correlation between exposure of infants to low concentrations of PCBs and dioxin to weakened immunity because of suppressed levels of disease-fighting white blood cells.

And what about chemicals and other pollutants that act as hormone disrupters?

There is growing concern about pollutants that can act as hormone disrupters, which cause growth, weight, brain, and behavioral disorders. Numerous studies indicate that extremely low levels of hormone disrupters can adversely affect developing embryos, human fetuses, and infants less than six months old.

So far 51 chemicals, many of them widely used, have been shown to act at extremely low levels as hormone disrupters in wildlife, laboratory animals, and some populations of humans. Examples include:

- Dioxins: dioxins occur when chlorine containing compounds are incinerated producing the infamous chlorinated hydrocarbons. These ashes settle to earth and form dioxins.
- PCBs: PCBs are a group of chlorinated hydrocarbons widely distributed in the environment and capable of being biologically magnified in the food chain.
- Various chemicals which occur in plastics
- Pesticides
- Lead and mercury

Environmental chemicals and other toxins: A massive problem still little understood.

Why do we know so little about the harmful effects of chemicals?

According to risk assessment expert Joseph V. Rodricks, *"Toxicologists know a great deal about a few chemicals, a little about many, and next to nothing about most."* The US National Academy of Sciences estimates that only about 10% of the nearly 100,000 chemicals in commercial use have been thoroughly screened for toxicity and only 2% have been adequately tested to determine whether they are carcinogens, teratogens, or mutagens. Carcinogens cause cancer, teratogens cause birth defects, and mutagens cause random genetic mutations in our cellular DNA. Hardly any of these chemicals have been screened for damage to the nervous, endocrine, and immune systems.

Each year we introduce into the marketplace about 1,000 new chemicals about whose potentially harmful effects we have little knowledge. Currently about 99.5% of the commercially used chemicals in the United States are not regulated by our federal and state governments.

There are three major reasons for this lack of information. *First*, under existing laws most chemicals are considered innocent until proven guilty. No one is required to investigate whether they are harmful. *Second*, there are not enough funds, personnel, facilities and test animals to provide such information for more than a small fraction of the many chemicals we encounter in our daily lives. *Third*, even if we could make a reasonable estimate of the biggest risks associated with particular technologies or chemicals (a very difficult and expensive thing to do) we know little about their possible interactions with other technologies and chemicals or about the effects of such interactions on human health and ecosystems. For example, just to study the possible different three-chemical interactions among the top 500 most widely used industrial chemicals would require 20.7 million experiments; a physical and financial impossibility.

The difficulty and expense of getting information about the harmful effects of chemicals is one reason an increasing number of environmentalists and health officials are pushing for much greater emphasis on *pollution prevention*. This strategy greatly reduces the need for statistically uncertain and controversial toxicity studies and exposure standards. It also reduces the risk posed by potentially hazardous chemicals and products and their possible but poorly understood multiple interactions. (G. Tyler Miller, Jr. and Associates, eds., *Living in the Environment*, 11th ed. [Brooks-Cole Publishing: 2000], 17: 436-444)

What this article means to me is that what we know about harmful man-made chemicals is only the tiniest tip of a very big iceberg. What this article means to me is that if we are serious about our health and the health of those we love, we must become more proactive in protecting the quality of the sources of our food, water, and air. Organic standards

Section 3 - Optimizing Results

have been in place in some areas of our food supply now for over thirty years. "Buying organic" is one way to ensure food safety and food quality. Making sure you have an effective point-of-use drinking water purifier for your drinking and cooking water is also essential. If the chlorine content of your water is high, then you should also invest in a system that filters bath and shower water too. Pay attention to air quality reports wherever you live. Make sure you are not suffering from "sick building syndrome" and if necessary, get an effective air purifier for your home, office and car. Lastly, you must inspect your household cleaning supplies, gardening supplies, and personal care products like shampoo, deodorant and toothpaste. Hazardous chemicals and additives have found their way into everything. Organic standards are the best way to prevent these substances from invading and adversely affecting your hearth and home and body. (RM)

How to Find Certified Organic Foods

How to find Certified Organic Foods is easy. I just went to www.google.com and did a simple web search on the words: *certified organic foods*. Hundreds of sources were listed. *Why* to find and use Certified Organic Foods is also easy. Certified Organic Foods are the healthiest, cleanest, most nutritious and most pollutant-free foods available. The certified organic farmer or grower understands the connection between mineral-rich soil and nutrient-rich food crops. No pesticides, herbicides, fungicides; no artificial ingredients, colorings, preservatives, additives; no genetic manipulation or crossing species; no antibiotics or hormones; no premature harvesting and artificial ripening of plants; no inhumane treatment of animals—just the food, the whole food and nothing but the food. For a list of your local organic growers go to www.csa.com

Each Cell Is a Factory

In order to function properly, each cell in our body has very specific requirements in terms of raw materials. These nutrient raw materials enable each cell to perform its specific metabolic task. As a result of healthy metabolism, each cell produces beneficial products *and each cell also produces waste products that are detrimental and toxic to that same cell.*

These toxic waste products must be identified, neutralized, and eliminated on a regular basis *or the cell will get sick, degenerate and die.* If the cell replicates (divides or gives birth to offspring cells) in a condition of unresolved toxicity or unrepaired damage, or if it is weak, sick, or diseased, it will pass on these *irregularities* to the offspring cells. This situation can lead to the continuous replication of abnormal or irregular cells within tissues and organs of the body. This is simply one way for a degenerative disease process to manifest (including cancers).

Vigilant quality control in the form of conscientious monitoring of the incoming raw materials and the outgoing products and waste products of our little cellular factories is, metaphorically speaking, one of the keys to health. When cells are healthy the symptoms of health are manifesting in abundance, physical energy, mental clarity, good moods, better digestion, no aches and pains.

When cells are not healthy, the symptoms of cellular dis-ease begin to manifest: fatigue, aches and pains, inattention, confusion, depression, mood swings, indigestion, and others. The cells of our body are constantly sending messages to the cells of our brain to make sure the brain is aware of how all the little factories are doing. Think of the brain as the inspector general for all those trillion plus factories. Are we listening? Are we in communication with the inspector general in our own body/brain/mind? How do we respond to the various calls we get on a daily basis from the cells to the *inspector general*? How are we communicating with our own internal cellular communication network?

Each Cell is a Factory

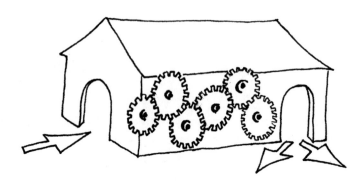

Raw Materials	Beneficial Products	Waste Products
Food	Normal Metabolism	Urine
Water	Energy and Vitality	Feces
Oxygen Inhaled	Balance and Harmony	Perspiration
Environmental Toxins	Homeostasis	Carbon Dioxide Exhaled
	Biomodulation	Metabolic Toxins

Section 3 - Optimizing Results

According to Our Factory Metaphor How Do We Stay Healthy?

1. Choose only the highest quality raw materials for fuel, repair and building supplies. This is the area of *diet and nutrition* and involves all the *complementary* and/or *insulting* habits we have in the interconnected areas of food selection and storage, meal planning and preparation, chewing and digestion, transit time and elimination.

2. Maintain the balance between the incoming raw materials and the outgoing products and waste products. This is the area of movement and rest and exercise. Exercise includes all the vital habits that together join forces to deliver nutrients to the cells and carry waste from the cells and out of the body. Movement and rest, proper breathing and hydration, bending and stretching our skeletal muscles, proper chewing and peristalsis (the proper moving of the intestinal muscles) and digestion, transit time and elimination. All the various nutrients and toxins make their way into our cells and are carried away from our cells (once properly identified and neutralized) primarily through the active circulation of blood and lymph. Our blood circulates in very well-defined channels of arteries, veins and capillaries, with the heart muscles being the activating pump responsible for proper circulation. **Please take note: We have twice as much lymphatic fluid in our body than blood; and there is no lymphatic pump equivalent to the heart.** Lymphatic fluids contain lymphocytes which are the cells that make up the major constituents of our Immune System. The primary purpose and most important reason to exercise regularly is to make sure you are effectively circulating your lymphatic fluid.

In other words: **You are the pump for your lymphatic fluid.** No matter how well you eat and drink, **if you do not exercise**; you do not move your lymphatic fluid. If you do not move your lymphatic fluid effectively, than you are not succeeding in delivering all the nutrients to all your cells and you are not succeeding in carrying all those toxic wastes away from your cells. You do not have to become an fitness champion or martial artist or marathon runner. You just have to move regularly.

3. Exercise vigilant quality control of the factory. This is the area of **mindfulness**. This is the area of **personal responsibility**. This is where the value of being **proactive** in your own self-education and self-care really shows up. You are not only the **Inspector General** for all those trillion plus cellular factories, you are the boss, the CEO: the buck stops with you. So, extending our factory metaphor just a little bit longer: What kind of CEO of your own body do you want to be? Some suggestions: Do only what serves to produce the most desirable products and waste products from your factory. Make responsible, ecological choices every day. (Reduce, reuse and recycle whenever possible.) Be fully present at all times to nourish, strengthen, and acknowledge everyone and every thing that contributes to the health and well-being of the factory. Implement innovative proposals and ideas. Reward all complementary habits. Consistently praise every factory worker at every level, every day for their tireless and awe-inspiring work ethic: 24–7–365 throughout your entire life. Gratitude is one of the keys to proactive health.

Section 3 - Optimizing Results

🌰 Phase One Foods

The easiest and most effective way to approach Phase One of your *Intestinal Regeneration Program* is to understand that Phase One is temporary (not permanent) and primarily designed to calm down and quiet down your entire digestive system. Why? To make healing possible. To make the miracle of physical regeneration more likely to occur. There is unfortunately a lot of disagreement about which foods are conducive to normal digestive function and which foods should be avoided if you are symptomatic. It's difficult trying to make perfect sense of all the sources of disagreement. Each dietary perspective has its basis for its various suggestions. My suggestions come from my own experiences and from the experiences of many others over the past forty years. All the great results and inspiring stories from my clients that you have read about came from following this *Intestinal Regeneration Program* as it has been described in these pages. The following list of foods is the most complementary during Phase One. If it is not on the following list, I advise you to avoid it during Phase One.

During Phase One, I do not advocate the use of any raw food, fresh fruit, fruit juice, or vegetable juice. All the foods listed below should be properly cooked: not over cooked, properly cooked. Grains should be boiled or pressure-cooked. Vegetables should be made into soup, or steamed, boiled, sautéed, or baked. The simplest forms of cooking should be used during Phase One. Your only beverages should be water and salt and the broth from your soups. Here is a list of the most beneficial foods during Phase One:

Cooked whole cereal grains for porridge: short grain brown rice, whole oats, whole barley; sea vegetables alone or in soups: kombu, wakame, arame, hijiki, dulse; root vegetables: onions, carrots, turnips, parsnips, daikon radish, burdock root, leeks; land vegetables: broccoli, cauliflower, brussel sprouts, celery, cabbage, corn, peas, string beans, snowpeas, squash. There are several varieties of squash that are extremely helpful during Phase One. Please try all of these: butternut, buttercup, hubbard, hokaido, acorn. Steamed greens make a tasty and nutritious side dish. Wash, cut, and lightly steam your greens. You can add some tamari soy sauce to enhance the flavor: kale, collards, parsley, watercress, broccoli rabe, carrot tops, chicory, chinese cabbage, bok choy, dandelion greens, mustard greens, turnip greens, scallions. Miso soup before meals is also fine.

Please take note: The strictness of your adherence to my suggestions for your Phase One foods is really up to you and your accurate assessment of your current intestinal condition and disorder. If you grade yourself on a scale of 1–10, 1 being a state of optimal digestive health and 10 being hospitalized for your condition, anyone grading themselves 6 or above should follow the strictest guidelines for Phase One for best results. If you grade yourself 1–5, my advice to you is to follow my Phase One Foods Simplified suggestions from page 141.

Section 3 - Optimizing Results

Reflective Practice

This essay was written by one of my clients, Bob Dufresne, PhD. I've included it here because it captures the essence of one of the most important habits for anyone attempting to be more proactive in their own self-care, self-reflection. RM

In my attempts to improve my health through better nutrition, I have become aware of certain deficiencies in my lifestyle that go well beyond physical nutrients. The starting point for this awareness comes from the dynamic principle at the heart of functional nutrition: *that nothing is neutral.* Everything, as it turns out, is either complementary or insulting to the way our body has been designed to function. Complementary habits allow and encourage the body to do what it was made to do thereby leading to a healthy state. Insulting habits interrupt, impair and interfere with the natural mechanisms of the body, thereby leaving the body in a vulnerable state; a state more likely to invite disease.

When faced with this simple principle whose merits one can easily prove to oneself, a troubling question arises: Why would anyone choose insulting habits over complementary habits? Even when we are given the appropriate information and hold the very best of intentions, we often fail to do what is complementary to our own bodies. For me part of the answer lies in the word, "habit." Complementary habits are habits only when you have incorporated them into your life in such a way that other parts of your life reinforce your consistent practice of those habits. But how does this come about? This is truly the most difficult part. We cannot merely go through our lives following our old habits. We must engage in a serious conversation with our *selves*. We must engage in what I like to call *reflective practice*.

Reflective practice means we must raise our actions to a level of awareness where we can exert control over those actions. We must become fully conscious about how the complementary actions we choose will improve our lives. We must see how the complementary actions we take are also complementary with other aspects of our life. In order to see these things we must stop the wheels of perpetual motion and busyness in our lives and reflect deeply upon the simplest things, including what we eat and how we eat. We must come to certain conclusions about how our decisions in this most basic area of life have enormous repercussions in all the other areas of our life. Everything else we do in life, we can do better when we have our physical health as our foundation.

In coming to this realization I have become aware that my own lifestyle leaves very little time for reflective practice. I would like to observe that this seems to be a common ailment among many who live in this modern world of ours. I have come to the conclusion that to live "a healthy life" in all aspects of life, we must work towards the goal of making this most central complementary habit, reflective practice, the most important complementary habit of all.

Bob Dufresne, PhD, June 18, 2004
The University of Massachusetts Physics Education Research Group

Section 3 - Optimizing Results

🌰 Some Essential Information About Salt

This article comes from the Winter 2004 newsletter of The Grain and Salt Society. I have edited this article liberally. RM

Archeological findings dating back to 700 BC link the Celts to the craft of salt mining and sea salt harvesting. Earlier writings talk about the salt trade around the world. The Egyptians, Greeks, Romans, Chinese and many more all relied on salt. Their diets, and in some cases, their politics and economies centered around salt.

Salt is actually a chemical term for a substance produced by a reaction of an acid with a base. The terms "salt" and "sodium" are used interchangeably, but technically this is not correct. "Salt" is sodium chloride. By weight, it is 40% sodium and 60% chloride. Sodium is an essential nutrient, a mineral that the body cannot manufacture itself, but one which is required for life and good health. Human blood contains 0.9% sodium chloride, or salt; the same concentration as found in hospital IV solutions. Our body needs salt, and the trace minerals that come along for the ride with naturally occurring sea salt. Without these minerals and trace minerals in the blood and lymph, tissues and cells, the body quickly loses the ability to maintain *homeostasis*. When homeostasis is threatened, the door is flung wide open for the full spectrum of symptoms representing all the degenerative disease processes to begin.

Mineral salts create electrolytes. Electrolytes, often called *the sparks of life*, are the substances that carry electrical currents and impulses throughout the body. Electrolytes carry biochemical messages to the cells in the organs that make up all the systems of the body. When electrolytes are low, communication slows down. When biochemical communication slows down, sickness and disease begin. Electrolytes are also necessary for enzyme production. Enzymes are biochemical *catalysts* for all metabolic functions. Enzymes are responsible for digesting food, for absorbing nutrients, for muscle function, for hormone function and much more. Our biological need for salt that contains a balance of naturally occurring minerals and trace minerals (as found in the Celtic sea salt) is very real. These minerals get used up in a trillion metabolic activities and must be replenished on a regular, daily, and continual basis to maintain health and well-being.

It is true that we need salt to live. Our own cellular makeup is very similar to that of sea water. The pH of sea water and the pH of human blood are almost identical. Much more than a mere solution of salt water, the ocean's waters contain a varied and complex combination of minerals and trace minerals. These facts have made salt a very precious commodity in human societies the world over for thousands of years.

Animals will travel miles for salt. It is no coincidence that some of the early travel routes wound and meandered to include locations of natural salt licks. A primordial appetite for salt has driven man and animal alike. Its natural occurrence in the oceans, soil and in our veins, explains our natural desire for salt. While today's most prevalent condiment may not conjure up images of empires and revolutions, the health and well-being of the past and present peoples has been and continues to be determined by salt.

Salt is a mineral and the only non-biological food that humans eat routinely. It is also interesting to note that water is the only non-biological liquid that humans drink.

A healthy active lifestyle demands sufficient salt intake. Human life is dependent on the presence of sodium in the blood and body fluids. Sodium, in the form of sodium chloride plays an important part in the primary activities of digestion and absorption of nutrients. Salt activates the first digestive enzyme *salivary amylase*, which is responsible for the breakdown of all carbohydrates. Sodium chloride is used to make hydrochloric acid, essential for all the digestive activity which happens in the stomach. Sodium functions best when other minerals and trace minerals are present. In naturally occurring Celtic sea salt, calcium, magnesium, potassium, and about 40 other minerals and trace minerals are all present.

Nutritional science has always isolated minerals to determine their usefulness but it is now clear that a full spectrum and large variety of

Section 3 - Optimizing Results

minerals in trace amounts is more important to human health than mega amounts of only a few minerals. This last sentence has relevance when it comes to taking nutritional supplements too. A supplement containing a full-spectrum of micro-nutrients, even in trace amounts is more helpful to the body than single or isolated nutrients in mega amounts.

The Negative Impacts of Cold Foods and Beverages

Our internal body temperature is 98.6 degrees. That's pretty hot. Our body works very hard twenty-four hours a day to maintain our internal temperature at this number. A few degrees warmer and we have a fever. A fever usually occurs as a response of the immune system to some kind of invading virus or bacteria. As our blood and body temperatures rise, the speed of our circulating immune cells increases dramatically. *A well-nourished body doesn't make mistakes.* If you have been healthy and you suddenly get a fever, there is a good reason for it. Your body is trying to protect you and defend you from something trying to make you sick. It is always best to understand why the body does what it does, so that we can cooperate with it, rather than suppress and punish it. In very rare cases, the body simply cannot handle the toxic burden of the invading organism or infection and the fever goes too high. At this point medical intervention is necessary.

On the cooler side of 98.6 degrees is a condition called hypothermia. Once hypothermia sets in, the body will automatically start to shiver and shake in a desperate attempt to heat itself up and keep the circulation of blood and lymph flowing. If hypothermia persists, the body will lose its ability to function normally and the person will require emergency medical intervention or die. These are extreme examples but are illustrative of the main point. Heating up our body increases circulation and cooling down our body decreases circulation. One of the oldest and wisest definitions of sickness from various natural healing traditions comes down to one word: blockage. Consequently, one of the oldest and wisest remedies in all the natural healing traditions is *restoring circulation* or *increasing circulation*. One of the best forms of proactive prevention is to maintain healthy levels of circulation by doing nothing that will cause any internal *blockages*.

The most obvious type of blockage is with our blood and lymph. Cold foods, beverages and influences tend to shock the body and then block the flow of many things: blood, lymph, thoughts, feelings, energy. These shocks and blocks can also affect the flow of water and nutrients into our cells (tissues, muscles, bones) and the flow of waste products out of our cells. These kinds of shocks and blocks can also slow down and inhibit the essential metabolic activities going on inside of cells. Eating foods, drinking beverages, eating snacks, taking supplements, wearing clothes and engaging in various activities that complement and support the body's ability to maintain its normal internal temperature are among the most important things we can do to regain our health and maintain our health. Anything we do to shock or block this normal internal temperature literally pushes us and our body in the direction of sickness and disease.

One of the most insulting habits in America today is the habit of drinking ice-water. Drinking ice-water before a meal shocks the stomach and blocks the release of all the normal digestive juices. This can result in the rapid onset of indigestion and heartburn and if not corrected, can and will eventually lead to the full range of IBS–IBD symptoms. Drinking cold orange juice first thing in the morning is a habit performed daily by millions and millions of people. If you are currently experiencing digestive system problems, they will not get better until you stop this habit of ice-cold beverages.

In over thirty years of my nutrition counseling experience I have met with and talked to dozens and dozens of women with ovarian cysts and uterine fibroids, PMS, and irregular periods to name only a few common complaints. In every case, there was the habit of eating and drinking cold foods and beverages; especially ice-water. The biggest problem with ice cream is not the dairy or sugar or fat. The biggest problem with ice cream is the coldness. Children say they love those iced *slushies* and *slurpee* drinks, but they wreck havoc on digestion and can cause constipation, headaches, allergies and behavioral problems. Why? The effect of the coldness shuts down normal digestion, slows down circulation and blocks the flow of normal metabolism everywhere in the body. The body experiences cold foods and beverages as a shock and these kinds of shocks are extremely insulting to the body. If it only occurred once in a great while, the body would recover. Unfortunately, cold foods and beverages are the normal tendency today, not the exception. Eliminating this insulting habit is one of the fastest ways to initiate a process of intestinal regeneration.

Some Thoughts on Acid and Alkaline Food Balances

The subject of internal pH balances of our blood, lymph, saliva, urine, and cellular fluids is of critical importance in the conversation about how foods, beverages, supplements, medications, and all other influences affect our health. The subject of acid-alkaline influences is one of the most important and one of the most controversial. I am interested in introducing you to some basic concepts in this book and I encourage you to check my website for more complete explanations in the future. www.healingdigestiveillness.com

The term pH refers to the presence of hydrogen ions detectable in a solid or liquid. For health purposes the solids and liquids of importance include our foods and beverages and how they are affecting our internal body fluids, organs, bones, systems and cells. The more hydrogen ions that are present in something, the more acid that something is. The fewer hydrogen ions that are present, the more alkaline it is. The pH scale is a numerical reference that designates the relative alkalinity or acidity of something using the numbers from 0 to 14: 0 being the most acid, 14 being the most alkaline.

The pH of normal, healthy human blood falls in the very narrow range of 7.35 to 7.45. Our body works very hard all the time to maintain the pH of our blood at this level and within this range. Everything we eat and drink, take as a supplement, and take as a medication affects the pH of our blood and other internal fluids. Physical activity affects pH. Stress affects pH. Sleep and rest affect pH. The steady maintenance of the proper pH levels of all of our internal body fluids (but especially our blood and lymph) is one of the most important biomodulating activities our bodies perform 24–7–365. When we talk about the miracle of *homeostasis*, the regulation of our internal pH balances is one of the most important miracles there is.

A quick check of any anatomy and physiology textbook will tell us that with the exception of the hydrochloric acid produced by our stomach, most other fluids in the body are alkaline: the blood and lymph, saliva, bile salts, urine. Metabolic waste products from normal cellular activity are all acid waste products and need to be eliminated on a regular and continual basis. Our bones are a huge storehouse of alkaline reserves. Our bones are composed primarily of the very alkaline minerals of calcium, sodium, and potassium. If we consume too many foods and beverages that are acid-forming our body has no choice but to steal alkaline minerals from the bones. This is one of the leading causes of osteoporosis. Cholesterol is an alkaline material produced by the liver to protect the lining of our arteries from blood that may be too acidic after the consumption of too many acid-forming foods and beverages. These are just two examples, but clearly you can see that knowing which foods and beverages help our body to maintain normal pH balances is critical to our health and well-being. It is also a critical point to understand (perhaps the most critical of all), that *a well-nourished body doesn't make mistakes*. Any symptom of dis-ease that shows up in the body is a direct message about persistent insulting habits and influences in our dietary and lifestyle choices.

One of the outstanding benefits of the watercure recipe is its constant alkalinizing effect. The presence of organic sea salt in our drinking water helps to maintain the proper pH balances of our blood and lymph, and helps to eliminate the normal acid wastes from the metabolic activities of organs and cells. Freshly cooked whole foods that have been grown in mineral-rich soils are the best foods to maintain proper pH levels. The other Phase One food choices in our *Intestinal Regeneration Program* are also designed to address our core acid-alkaline balances (that is, to avoid acid-forming influences and include more alkalinizing influences). This is why I am suggesting the watercure, miso soup, cooked whole grain porridge, sea vegetables, and other cooked vegetables. Processed foods in general all have an acid-forming impact on the body. You rarely hear of anyone suffering an illness from taking in too many alkaline forming foods and beverages. However, you constantly hear about foods and beverages that are too acid-forming. Here is a short list of some of the commonly used (and abused) acid-forming foods and beverages in the Standard American Diet (SAD):

Section 3 - Optimizing Results

Coffee, tea, wine, beer, spirits (ie any form of alcohol), fruit juice (yes, that includes orange juice, grape juice and apple juice), refined cane sugar, chocolate, honey, maple syrup, Equal, Aspartame, Nutrasweet, all soft drinks, sodas and carbonated beverages, almost all processed and pre-packages breakfast cereals (especially all those instant oatmeal type things), most commercial flour-butter-sugar combinations (bread, pastries, donuts, bagels, muffins, cookies, cakes, pies, waffles, pancakes, pop-tarts), processed meats (salami, bologna, pepperoni, sausages), most commercial salad dressings and tropical and semi-tropical fruits and fruit juices like oranges, grapefruit, bananas, pineapples, mangoes, papaya, etc. Even certain vegetables of tropical origin like potatoes, tomatoes, and eggplant and vegetables containing high levels of oxalic acid like asparagus, spinach, and red beets are acid-forming. Unfortunately, this list contains many foods commonly consumed by millions of people every day. Fortunately, we have discovered that many of these combinations are creating an internal environment that is not allowing the digestive system to restore normal functioning.

Here is a list of pH evaluations of certain foods and beverages. This information comes from the book *Acid and Alkaline* by Herman Aihara. Keep in mind that cooking can alter the pH of food.

Stomach acid: 1.5
Red wine: 3.5
Beer: 4.5
Cow's milk: 6.5
Human saliva: 7.1
Human blood: 7.4   (7.35-7.45)
Ocean water: 8.1
Pancreatic juice: 8.8   (aka "bile")
Lye soap: 9.1
Baking soda: 12.0

Section 3 - Optimizing Results

pH values of some common foods: from most acid to most alkaline
pH value: name of food:

1.9	limes	5.0	pumpkin
3.3	lemons	5.1	carrots
3.4	cranberries	5.2	beets
2.9	plums	5.2	squash
2.9	vinegar	5.3	cabbage
3.0	soda	5.4	turnips, spinach
3.1	apples	5.5	beans, sweet potatoes
3.1	apple cider	5.6	asparagus
3.1	fruit jams and jellies	5.7	cheese
3.2	grapefruit	5.8	potatoes
3.3	strawberries	6.0	wheat flour
3.4	blackberries, raspberries	6.0	tuna fish
3.5	oranges, peaches	6.1	peas
3.6	cherries	6.2	salmon
3.7	apricots	6.3	butter, corn, dates
3.8	pears	6.4	oysters
4.0	grapes	6.5	cow's milk
4.2	tomatoes	6.9	shrimp
4.5	beer	7.0	pure water
4.6	bananas	7.5	sea salt

Why Use Supplemental Digestive Enzymes?

This brief article may also appear in other places under the title: "The Law of Adaptive Secretion of Enzymes." This information is culled from the work of two of the world's foremost experts on supplemental digestive enzymes: Dr. Edward Howell and Viktoras Kulvinskas.

One question that often gets asked is this: If I use supplemental digestive enzymes, will it inhibit my own body's ability to produce its own? In other words, there is a concern that by taking supplemental digestive enzymes, we are somehow making the body lazy and thereby undermining our future health and vitality in the process.

Nothing could be further from the truth. *According to The Law of Adaptive Secretion of Digestive Enzymes*, first described by research physiologists at Northwestern University:

> "The amount of digestive enzymes secreted by the pancreas in response to carbohydrate, protein, and fat in the diet (per meal) was measured and it was found that the strength of each enzyme varied with the amount of each of the materials it was required to digest."

Later it is stated:

> "*The Law of Adaptive Secretion of Digestive Enzymes* holds that the organism values its enzymes highly and will make no more than are needed for the job. If some of the food is digested by enzymes in the food, the body will make less concentrated enzymes."

> "*The Law of Adaptive Secretion of Digestive Enzymes* has been confirmed by dozens of university laboratories throughout the world."

"If the human organism must devote a huge portion of its enzyme potential to making digestive enzymes, it spells trouble for the whole body because there is a strain on the production of metabolic enzymes and there may not be enough enzyme potential to go around."

"If humans take more exogenous (outside) digestive enzymes as nature ordained, the enzyme potential will not have to waste so much of its heritage digesting food. It can distribute more of this precious commodity to the metabolic enzymes, where it rightfully belongs. This rightful distribution of enzyme energy will not only act to maintain health and prevent disease, but is expected to help cure established disease. The old saying that nature will cure really refers to metabolic enzyme activity, because there is no other mechanism in the body to cure anything."

These excerpts are from the book: *Enzyme Nutrition: The Food Enzyme Concept* by Dr. Edward Howell.

Please take note that this book was published in 1985, when Dr. Howell was 87 years old. It is now more politically correct to use the word "heal" instead of "cure" within natural healing circles. RM

"The length of life is inversely proportional to the rate of exhaustion of the enzyme potential of an organism. The increased use of food enzymes promotes a decreased rate of exhaustion of the enzyme potential." The Enzyme Nutrition Axiom formulated by Dr. Edward Howell.

The moral of our story? "Don't Dine Without Supplemental Digestive Enzymes!"

References for this article:

Dr. Edward Howell, *Enzyme Nutrition*, Avery Publishing Group, 1985

Victor P. Kulvinskas, *Don't Dine Without Enzymes*, L.O.V.E. Foods, 1994

Uses of Digestive Enzymes

Purify Blood: Is it possible that an enzyme can clean up and purify the blood? When you look at it from the simplest perspective, it makes sense. It is known that fungal forms, parasites, and bacteria are made up of proteins. Also, consider that the shell that protects a virus in our bodies is in fact a protein coating. The enzyme protease breaks down proteins. Could it be possible that ingesting protease on an empty stomach would help by breaking down undesirable organisms? An empty stomach is suggested since protease would then not have to be held in the digestive system to digest any protein foods that had been recently eaten, but freed up to enter the bloodstream and go after undesirable organisms and undigested food particles.

Strengthen the Immune System: Enzymes deliver nutrients, carry away toxic wastes, digest food, purify the blood, deliver hormones by feeding and fortifying the endocrine system, balance cholesterol and triglyceride levels, feed the brain, and cause no harm to the body. These factors contribute to the strengthening of the immune system.

Breakdown Fats: The enzyme lipase breaks down and digests fats. When added to your meal as a supplement, it is able to do this job in the digestive tract. This takes stress off the gall bladder, liver and pancreas. When taken between meals, it will be stored in your liver and called upon when needed.

Lowers Cholesterol: Lipase may also help in lowering cholesterol

Take Off Excess Weight and Fat: Many overweight people have metabolic imbalances. The endocrine system is a critical component of our whole metabolism. Once we are able to fortify the endocrine system, get the bowels working regularly, and digest our food rather than turning it into fat, we have a successful combination for losing weight. Rather than creating common "weight loss" which is nothing more than water loss (which is a form of dehydration!), we will instead burn fat and properly digest our food. This process is not instantaneous because we have to lose fat instead of weight. It takes longer but it is healthier and longer lasting. Best of all, it does no harm.

Improve Skin Quality: An adequate supply of enzymes is absolutely essential for keeping your skin young looking and healthy. According to researchers, Amber Ackerson and Anthony Cichoke in Portland, Oregon, enzymes fight the aging process by increasing the blood supply to the skin, bringing with it life-giving nutrients, and carrying away waste products that otherwise may make our skin look dull and wrinkled. Circulation slows down as we get older. Eating a diet with raw fruits and vegetables, which is enzyme rich, and taking a complete enzyme supplement becomes important with age.

Enhance Mental Capacity: Your body uses glucose called from the liver to feed and fortify the hypothalamus. This long-lasting glucose is made from protein stored in the liver. All plant enzymes are amino acids, which come from protein foods. Our red blood cells do the work of carrying oxygen to our brain. Nutrients have to be delivered throughout our body by means of the enzyme delivery system. When this is not accomplished, we become fatigued and are less able to think clearly. Remember that the hypothalamus directs our endocrine system and is responsible for water balance, body temperature, appetite, and even emotions.

Cleanse the Colon: Undigested foods that are stored in the colon began with a digestive problem. In the colon, undigested protein will putrefy; starch, sugars, and other carbohydrates will ferment and fats will turn rancid. If we eat more than one meal per day, we should experience at least two bowel movements per day to rid our body of these toxins. Enzyme supplements along with vital probiotics, aid in natural colon functioning and regularity.

Enhance Sleep: Nutrients that are able to get past the brain's barrier create insomnia and depression (this refers to undigested food particles not the proper delivery of micronutrients). The undernourished endocrine system may create a malfunction in our hormonal system, which can upset our nervous system and sleep patterns. However, if we are able to correctly digest our food and deliver nutrients to keep the endocrine system and nervous system in balance, then we can regain normal sleep functions easily.

References for this article:

Dr. Edward Howell, *Enzyme Nutrition*, Avery Publishing Group, 1985

Victor P. Kulvinskas, *Don't Dine Without Enzymes*, L.O.V.E. Foods, 1994

Why Probiotic Supplements Are So Important

The word probiotics means *for life*. Probiotics refers to a class of beneficial bacterial organisms that live inside our bodies, primarily in our digestive systems, which provide us with an astonishing variety of important health benefits. These bacteria, like the bacteria that live outside of our bodies, represent a complex interdependent web of life. This web of beneficial bacteria is often referred to as our internal microflora, our inner ecology, the human microbiome and often quite simply as the garden within.

> You often hear about *ecology*, the relationship between organisms and their environment. Within your body there is an entire miniature ecosystem, a microecology, which has a major influence on your health. This inner ecology is made up of the *microflora*, more than 400 species of microscopic living bacteria, creating an internal environment that is diverse, complex, interrelated, and ever-changing. This population, although minute, is so enormous that the number of beneficial bacterial cells in our body at any one time (when we are healthy that is) is greater than the total number of all the other cells in our body. The *microflora* are essential to our well-being. These bacteria provide very real *beneficial* effects. They limit the populations of harmful bacteria. They assist in the process of digestion. They manufacture essential nutrients. When our gut ecology is in balance, we thrive. (Nigel Plummer, PhD, *Optimal Digestion*, [New York: Avon Books, 1999], 46)

Section 3 - Optimizing Results

A Brief History of Probiotics in the Human Diet

There is nothing new about beneficial bacteria in the human diet. For thousands of years cultures around the world have figured out ingenious ways to pickle and ferment various grains, beans, fruits, and vegetables. Beer, wine, yogurt, kefir, kimchi and miso are food products familiar to most of us today. These foods and many others like them are thousands of years old. The knowledge of the presence of harmful bacteria, which make up only one percent of all the known bacteria in existence, was not discovered until the early 1800s. For thousands of years human beings were exposed on a daily basis to a variety of bacteria in their environment, in their food, water, air, shelter and clothing. The modern emphasis on antibiotics has created the illusion that all bacteria are bad. This is simply not true. Our over-emphasis on sterile antiseptic environments has overshadowed the knowledge of beneficial bacteria. Today all of that is changing as we rediscover the many benefits of daily probiotic supplementation.

How Do Probiotics Affect Digestion?

Of the 400 or so strains of beneficial bacteria that have been found inside the human digestive system, two strains stand out. *Acidophilus* is the dominant probiotic working inside the small intestine and *bifidus* is the dominant probiotic working inside the large intestine. In this section we will focus on acidophilus and the small intestine. In the next section we will discuss bifidus and the large intestine. Probiotics affect digestion by assisting in the normal functioning of these organs.

What Happens Inside the Small Intestine?

The small intestine is a long, narrow, and when healthy, very flexible tube about half an inch to an inch in diameter and almost twenty-four feet long. It stretches from the pyloric valve of the stomach to the ileocecal valve (which sits at the junction between the small intestine and large intestine, where our appendix resides). It is composed of three sections, the duodenum, the jejunum, and the ileum. By the time our digested food reaches our small intestine, it should be completely broken down and in a liquid state. I say *should* because without proper chewing and plenty of supplemental digestive enzymes our food does not get completely broken down.

For the next six to twelve hours or so our liquefied food (called chyme) slides back and forth within well defined segments of the small intestine measuring three to six inches. The *gurgling sounds* we often hear soon after mealtimes is a result of this sliding and swooshing back and forth. Muscular contractions of the intestinal wall called peristalsis, move-the-chyme-along in a continuous and rhythmically forward motion. The primary purpose of this slow, methodical dance is to create the maximum amount of exposure to the millions and billions of finger-like projections protruding from every square inch of our small intestine lining, the villi and micro-villi. These villi perform one of the most important and miraculous functions of all. These villi reach out into the fertile soil of our completely digested meal and begin to extract the micro-nutrients into our blood. Tiny capillaries in the villi are linked to the hepatic vein which transports these nutrients to our liver for a final inspection, detoxification and storage. Without the direct assistance of acidophilus bacteria (and other beneficial bacteria in smaller amounts) by the trillions, this essential function of transformation and inner transportation of nutrients would not take place. It is not taking place normally inside the intestines of millions and millions of people today. Is it happening in you? Take probiotics every day and it will.

Cross Section of the Small Intestine

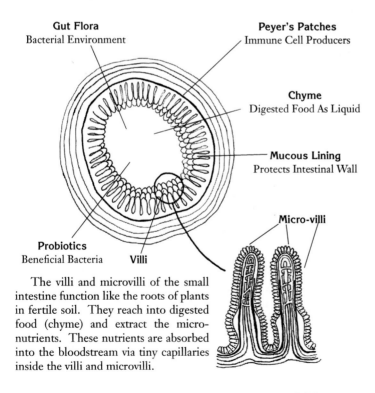

The villi and microvilli of the small intestine function like the roots of plants in fertile soil. They reach into digested food (chyme) and extract the micro-nutrients. These nutrients are absorbed into the bloodstream via tiny capillaries inside the villi and microvilli.

What Do the Acidophilus Bacteria Do?

Acidophilus bacteria by the trillions inhabit every square inch of our intestinal lining, the surface areas of the villi and micro-villi, and the tiny spaces between the villi, as well as permeate and infiltrate our liquefied food slush. Among many other benefits listed below, the acidophilus bacteria finalize the digestion of food particles, breaking them down into the smallest possible sizes, and then provide direct assistance in the mechanical transport to the surface of the micro-villi where absorption and assimilation into the bloodstream take place. When acidophilus bacteria do not exist in sufficient quantity or quality this miraculous nutrient transfer does not occur. This results in a condition called malabsorption syndrome. This condition adversely affects millions of North Americans today resulting in a very long list of uncomfortable symptoms from headaches, allergies and fatigue, to depression, constipation, and skin disorders, and many, many more.

The Benefits of Acidophilus:

Not all acidophilus is the same. The benefits listed below apply only to the DDS-1 strain of lactobacillus acidophilus produced by Nebraska Cultures. This is the only form of acidophilus that I use and recommend.

- Acidophilus bacteria help to maintain the proper pH balances throughout the entire gastro-intestinal tract. Much gas, cramping, and bloating can occur when the acid/alkaline balances are off.
- Acidophilus bacteria produce important digestive enzymes including lactase, protease and lipase. Lactase breaks down the sugar lactose found in milk, and all products made from milk; butter, cheese, yogurt. Protease breaks down proteins in both animal

and vegetable sources and lipase breaks down fats. When these enzymes are not present in sufficient quantities, the incomplete digestion of these foods results in bad breath, bloating, cramping, gas and general weakening of the intestine.

- Acidophilus bacteria produce acidophilin, a powerful natural antibiotic which inhibits the growth of pathogenic bacteria and opportunistic yeast infections like candida albicans.
- Acidophilus bacteria secrete B vitamins which are essential in completing the stages of digestion, absorption, and assimilation of nutrients, especially folic acid and B12.
- Acidophilus bacteria service and protect the many lymph nodes, called *Peyer's Patches* which line the small intestine. These lymph nodes are an essential part of our immune system and produce antibodies and release *natural killer cells* and other immune cells. This represents additional natural artillery that protects us from various kinds of invader organisms inside the gastrointestinal tract.

As if all of the above did not represent enough benefits, additional research by the scientists at *Nebraska Cultures* has revealed that the DDS-1 acidophilus may also:

- help reduce episodes of diarrhea and urinary tract and vaginal infections
- help reduce serum cholesterol levels
- help alleviate dermatitis and other skin disorders

Protecting the Garden Within

Now that we have a greater appreciation for some of the amazing health benefits we receive from supplemental probiotics like acidophilus, let's take a quick look at some of the harmful influences we can avoid and some of the helpful or complementary influences we can include in the rest of our diet and lifestyle:

Harmful influences include: antibiotics, alcohol, antacids, most prescription and over-the-counter drugs, all sources of caffeine, coffee, tea, soda, chlorine in our drinking or bathing water, chronic dehydration, lack of exercise, too much worrying, not enough sleep, overeating, too many carbonated beverages, processed foods in general, food additives, preservatives, colorings, enriching agents, bleaching agents, artificial sweeteners, flavor enhancers, excess dairy food consumption, excess meat and processed meat consumption, excess sugar in any form, exposure to environmental pollutants like solvents, cleaning agents, pesticides, herbicides, fungicides, eating or drinking anything too cold, eating late in the day, not chewing.

Helpful influences include: proper daily hydration, chewing our food, moderate daily exercise, enough sleep, stress management, meditation or yoga, open communication lines at home and at work, taking supplemental digestive enzymes, probiotics and superfoods like wild edible blue green algae, and all the other *habits of naturally healthy people*. Take one step at a time, one day at a time. Be and become more proactive in your own self-care. Get healthier and have more fun!

> The balance that exists among our microflora is an example of nature's incredible perfection. When microflora coexist in harmony, a healthy state of symbiosis results and we thrive. When they live not in symbiosis, but in dysbiosis, this disturbed inner ecology often results in a sense of unwellness or even disease.(Len Saputo, MD, *Optimal Digestion* [New York, Avon Books, 1999], 54)

The Importance of Bifidus

This section completes our three-part discussion about the important health benefits that result from a properly functioning digestive system. We have learned that avoiding insulting influences in the rest of our diet and lifestyle plays a role, practicing more complementary habits plays a role, and that supplemental digestive enzymes and probiotics, like acidophilus and bifidus also play important and essential roles. This section focuses on our amazing large intestine and how bifidus assists greatly in maintaining the health and proper functioning of this vital organ.

> The large intestine is so big, that it is connected to, touches, sits next to, or is in the vicinity of every major organ in the human body except the brain. Your colon touches most of your major blood vessels and nerves. A sluggish, poorly functioning colon can adversely affect any area of the body. (Richard Schulze, ND, *Healing Colon Disease Naturally*, [Santa Monica, CA, Natural Healing Publications], 35)

Health Begins or Ends in the Colon!

This phrase or something like it is very well known throughout the world of natural health and for good reason. A very high percentage of all the toxic waste removed from our cells, tissues, muscles, and organs ends up in the colon. The regular elimination of all this toxic material is one of the keys to health. The retention or re-absorption of any of this toxic material back into our body (a process known as autointoxication or self-poisoning) is a contributing factor in all forms of physical degeneration. Making sure our large intestine (or colon) is functioning properly is one of the most important things we could ever learn. Here are a few fundamentals.

What Happens Inside the Large Intestine?

By the time our digested food (chyme) reaches the colon, 90% or more of the nutrients have been absorbed and assimilated. The primary job of the large intestine is to accept our digested food as waste matter and to make sure it gets out of our body as fast as possible. Several factors must be functioning properly in order for this waste matter to be eliminated effectively. Proper hydration and water content, proper friendly bacteria (primarily bifidus), enough bulk and fiber, a healthy mucous lining, and effective peristalsis (the muscular contractions of the intestinal wall) must all be working together.

Let' go down inside the inner workings of our large intestine and take a closer look at what is supposed to be happening under ideal conditions:

The Normal Colon
colon is the term used to refer to the large intestine

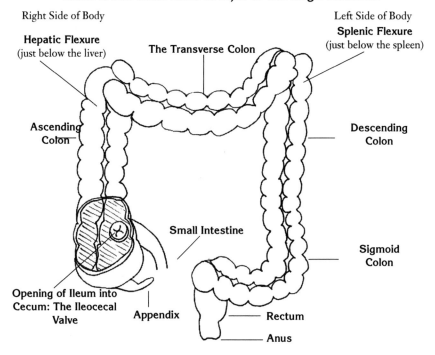

The small intestine and large intestine are connected by a valve called the ileo-cecal valve. The end part of the small intestine is called the ileum and the beginning part of the large intestine is called the cecum. If you know where your appendix is (lower right side of the abdomen, about two or three inches above the top of your hip bone in a straight line towards your navel), you've just located your ileo-cecal valve. Liquefied food (chyme) squirts through the fleshy opening of this valve and is immediately bathed with a variety of intestinal enzymes and friendly bacteria, mostly bifidus. In the cecum any excess water is utilized by the colon lining or reabsorbed into the body and what remains is highly toxic waste. Protecting the colon wall from this increasingly toxic waste matter is a layer of thick mucous composed of water and friendly bacteria. This mucous lining allows the proper degree of lubrication that in combination with regular muscular contractions (peristalsis) permits the smooth and rapid transit of waste removal.

The large intestine is about two to two and half inches wide, a round, fleshy, pouch-like tube. It is about five to six feet in length. Starting from the appendix area, the cecum moves up the right side of the abdomen towards the liver, where it turns to travel across the middle of the body (the transverse colon), crossing the spinal column at the L-5, S-1 location (between the fifth lumbar and first sacral vertebrae). When it reaches the left side of the body, near the spleen, it turns downward (descending colon), moving along the lower left side of the abdomen where it becomes the sigmoid colon (where it makes an s-like curve), then the rectum, then the anus. If everything is working properly, the time it takes for waste matter to enter and leave the colon should be between twelve to eighteen hours. It should take no longer than twenty-four hours for a meal we have just eaten to be thoroughly processed and eliminated from our body.

What Insults the Normal Functioning of the Colon?

Unfortunately the list is long. The large intestine, like all the parts and pieces of our gastro-intestinal tract, is a sensitive miniature eco-system much closer in design and function to a river or a garden than any kind of man-made machine. Often many of our dietary and lifestyle habits are mechanical and routine and simply do not take into account the simple organic nature of our anatomy and physiology. Here is a short list of some of the things that contribute to the toxic content of our waste matter on the one hand and slow down the normal functioning of our colon on the other:

Section 3 - Optimizing Results

Antibiotics, alcohol, antacids, all medications, coffee, tea, carbonated beverages, soda and diet sodas, chlorine in our drinking water, food additives, colorings, preservatives, pesticide, herbicide and fungicide residues, processed foods in general, especially products made from flour, butter, sugar and yeast, pasteurized dairy products, processed meats, over-cooking, over-eating, chronic unintentional dehydration, lack of exercise, and too much stress! (to name a few)

When bifidus and other probiotics, enzymes, and water are absent from this final and most important stage of elimination, the mucus lining of the large intestine becomes weak and sometimes disappears altogether. This situation causes the remaining fecal matter (waste) to become dry and hard. This causes the fecal transit time to slow down, allowing for unhealthy putrefaction and an increase in the production of pathogenic (bad) bacteria. This in turn can lead to the accumulation of fecal matter in the folds and pouches of the large intestine (haustra

The Abnormal Colon

colon is the term used to refer to the large intestine

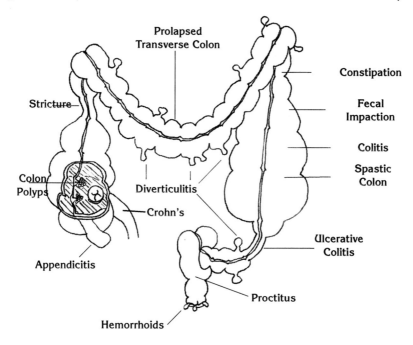

and diverticula). This unfortunate slow down and breaking down of normal functioning results in constipation. This results in many problems which all negatively affect our colon and the rest of our body too. These problems are usually lumped together under the name, Irritable Bowel Syndrome, or IBS.

What are the Benefits of Bifidus?

A healthy concentration of bifidus in the large intestine can help prevent the symptoms related to an irritable bowel, providing the following important benefits:

- Bifidus bacteria help to maintain the proper pH balances inside the large intestine. This balance is essential for normal functioning. When our pH is off, gas, cramping and bloating more easily occur.
- Bifidus bacteria serve as cofactors to various other beneficial bacteria, as well as to our food and digestive enzymes. This ensures thorough breakdown, prevents the formation of fecal plaque (hardened wastes), and increases colon transit time (which reduces the incidence of a sluggish bowel or constipation).
- Bifidus bacteria inhibit the growth of pathogenic bacteria by occupying the space that the pathogenic bacteria would use and through the release of natural and very powerful antibiotics.
- Bifidus bacteria live in and support the health of the mucous lining of the colon. It is the gradual weakening of this lining that accounts for a sluggish, constipated transit of waste material. This slowing down and holding on to our toxic waste creates many health problems.
- Bifidus bacteria service and protect the many lymph nodes that line the small and large intestine. These lymph-nodes are essential components of the human immune system and are currently the target of much research on the topic of gut-brain-immune connections.

Of course there is much more we can learn about the human digestive system and how best to nourish, cleanse and regenerate it. Always keep in mind that the two sides of the health coin play a role in all physical health problems and solutions:

1. Keeping toxins out of our body and getting them out effectively once already there.
2. Putting the very best nutrients into our body.

In these last three sections we have learned how important a healthy and normally functioning digestive system is. The nutrients for every cell and system in our body are absorbed and assimilated in our small intestine. Waste removal is the job of the large intestine. Whatever our food choices are, supplemental digestive enzymes will help to break those foods down and make the nutrients inside available to our body. Certain insulting habits need to be avoided or minimized and certain complementary habits need to be practiced and maintained.

Of all the processes essential to good health, proper elimination is certainly one of the most important. A healthy body depends upon a healthy bowel. The health of any tissue anywhere in the body depends upon the healthy tissue inside the large intestine. I am convinced and truly believe that most health problems begin more in the colon than any other part of the body. Health begins or ends in the colon! (Bernard Jensen, DC, ND, *Tissue Cleansing Through Bowel Management* [Escondido, CA: Bernard Jensen Publications, 1981], 35)

The Great American Pastime

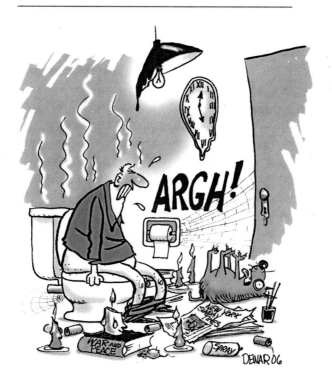

As usual, George has run out of reading material.

How to Expand Your Breakfast Menu

There is no doubt that breakfast is the most important meal of the day and that the rituals and habits you develop around this meal will have the biggest impact on you now, as you begin your *Intestinal Regeneration Program,* and later, as in the rest of your life! There is no doubt that one of the most insulting habits of people suffering from digestive system problems is the habit of eating late at night. For thousands of years most human beings did not have the luxuries of electricity, refrigerators, radio and televisions. People lived their lives according to the dictates of the seasons, the climate, their geography, the harvest, and most importantly, the rising and setting of the sun. People had to take advantage of the daylight hours to get their work done. Consequently they were usually up before dawn and in bed and fast asleep soon after sunset. Of course there were exceptions, but this is how it was for the most part, for thousands and thousands of years. Our bodies remember these habits. Our digestive system is still tied to these traditions and rhythms. One of the fastest ways to heal ourselves is to put ourselves back into accord with these old biological rhythms. Imagine that.

The word breakfast refers to the process of breaking the fast. To fast means to restrict ones intake of food. It could mean taking very little food to none at all. Sometimes the "fast" was voluntary and sometimes not. Traditionally, people did not have an excess of food hanging around, and they were very careful about eating only what was necessary and essential to stay healthy and get the work done. By the end of each winter season, it was common to fast from food entirely or to abstain from certain foods and influences. Sometimes this was

Section 3 - Optimizing Results

voluntary and sometimes it was absolutely necessary because the food supplies were either low or simply nonexistent. Today, people feel deprived if they are not eating something every five minutes. The first and most important physiological requirement for healing is rest and that would include resting the digestive system too.

The body never really rests, not completely. When it isn't digesting, it is able to direct its energy and resources to detoxification, cleansing and repair. If you practice the habit of not eating late at night, you will experience an acceleration of the healing process. What is *late at night?* It varies from person to person based on your current condition. Usually it means any time after sunset. The best way to find out what is going to work for you is to experiment.

During the mid 1990s, I had the good fortune of traveling to over 125 cities in the US and Canada for the purpose of teaching most of the health and nutrition fundamentals you are reading about in this book. I was amazed and delighted with the number of people who came up to me and shared stories about their grandparents and great-grandparents who ate very little at the evening meal and how they claimed that this was one of the secrets of their health and longevity. One of these people told me of a Russian saying attributed to some general: *Have breakfast by yourself. Have lunch with a friend. Give supper to your enemy!*

Traditionally, people ate more for breakfast and lunch and very little or nothing at all in the evening. I don't ask that anyone take my word for it on this or anything else I teach. The most important thing is to experiment. Find out what habits work best for you. Find out what habits are complementary and which ones are insulting. The other saying or proverb that has come down to us from our ancestors on this subject is this: king, prince, pauper. Eat like a king at breakfast, a prince at lunch, and a pauper at dinner. Try it.

I recommend that everyone experience at least a week or two of Phase One foods as I have described them on pages 141–155. Warm water and salt for your beverage and basic cooked whole grain porridge, miso soup, and steamed vegetables for your food. The sicker and weaker you are at the beginning the longer you may need to do this. Gradually, your uncomfortable digestive symptoms will subside, usually in three or four days. The first thing to add is miso soup. The next thing to add is steamed vegetable dishes. The next thing to add is small amounts of organic quality meat. I only advise this once you are having regular bowel movements and only if the meat is organic quality and only a small amount, usually no more than three or four ounces. Add ground chicken or turkey breast at first or perhaps some white meat fish. I do not advise adding any sweeteners or yogurt to your porridge. You must let the improving quality of your bowel movements and the condition of your intestines dictate when and how much you expand upon your most basic and simple breakfast routine; in other words, as you approach the golden banana status with your bowel movements on the one hand, and as you experience little to no intestinal gas, cramping, bloating, or discomfort on the other.

The next thing to add are side dishes of steamed greens: kale, collards, bok choy, chinese cabbage. You can add a dash of tamari to taste. Chew well. Fresh steamed greens are a great source of vitamins, minerals, and fiber. I do not advise using butter on your porridge. You can add small amounts of organic quality nut butters: peanut, almond, cashew. You can dry roast sunflower seeds, sesame seeds and walnuts and sprinkle these on your porridge, or eat them separately alongside your porridge. One of my favorite breakfast combinations is miso soup, steamed collard greens, and a porridge made with half-barley and half-oats with dry-roasted walnuts for a garnish. Mmm good!

Section 3 - Optimizing Results

🌰 What is Nutrigenomics?

"This new paradigm of health, which is now at our doorstep, that gives us the opportunity to revolutionize medicine and health-care is really based on a very simple notion and that notion is personalized medicine. It's about finding the right approach for each person based on their genes. This is what we call genomics. And specifically when it comes to food and nutrition, it's called nutri-genomics; which is the idea that food is actually information that talks to your genes and washes over your DNA and creates the outcome of your life which is either health or disease. And we have total control over that phenomena. We can actually control which (genetic) messages get turned on or turned off by exactly what we do to our bodies by what we eat. That's the power of nutrigenomics. That's the power of this new Health Model... this new Health Paradigm. I want you to understand that there are some basic laws of nature that you have to understand and follow to support your health. You need to consume foods that work with your genes and can contribute to an optimum functioning system. The fundamental concept behind Nutrigenomics is that everything you eat sends specific messages to your genes (which live inside the nucleus of your cells). Your genes, in turn, send messages to the regulatory or control centers of your body: your immune system, hormonal system, detoxification system, etc. These messages can be good messages like; "eliminate toxins" or "burn stored bodyfat" or "kill those bacteria I just inhaled through my nose" or they can be bad messages like: "make more LDL cholesterol" or "increase inflammation to my coronary arteries" or "slow down my brain function." The way food affects your genes is hard-wired and cannot be changed. But you have the ability to adapt to a nutrigenomics lifestyle that will turn on those messages of health (via optimal gene expression) by eating according to your body's natural instruction manual. In other words, nutrigenomics recognizes that food isn't just the stuff you put in your mouth that tastes good and fills you up. Food is actually information – it "talks" to your genes and washes over your DNA to create conditions of either health or disease, weight gain or weight loss, vitality or sluggishness. And you can control which messages get "turned on" or "turned off" through what you eat. The most influential thing you do every day is what (food) you put in your mouth. If we work with these basic core balances and provide the nutrients that restore normal functioning to our cells, and simply forget about diseases regardless of the disease; the body will heal and repair, restore, regenerate and revive. And that's the power of this Health Model: Functional Medicine, Functional Nutrition, Nutrigenomics…it's all the same thing based on the same natural principles and the same dietary and lifestyle practices. It's very exciting!"

Mark Hyman MD,

from his book/cd: **Nutrigenomics, How Food Talks to Your Genes to send Messages of Health or Disease.** *www.ultrawellnesscenter.com*

🌰 My Favorite Recipes for Phase One

Basic Miso Soup

Miso is a rich, fermented paste made from whole yellow soybeans or occasionally black soybeans, chickpeas, or aduki beans alone, or in combination with grains such as barley, brown rice, millet, and other grains. The whole beans and grains are combined with sea salt and natural koji, an enzyme-rich grain that starts the fermentation process. Used in Asia for thousands of year miso is an excellent aid in the production of healthy intestinal flora. It is rich in microorganisms and enzymes that strengthen the digestive enzymes and aid in the absorption and assimilation of nutrients in our foods. It also helps in the discharge of toxins from the body. It is high in protein, calcium, vitamin B, iron and other nutrients making it an essential food in every healthy whole foods kitchen. Miso can be used in grain, vegetable, fish and bean dishes, or in soups, homemade pickles, condiments, spreads, sauces, and as a medicine (for digestive upsets). Please experiment and discover the many uses of this wonderful health promoting food.

Ingredients and Directions

5 to 6 cups of spring or purified water (don't use tap water)
some wakame or kombu seaweed (sea vegetables)
1 large onion, sliced
1 large or two small carrots sliced
3 teaspoons of barley miso (sometimes called Mugi Miso) organic only
(Miso brands: Westbrae, Eden, Mitoku, South River, Miso Master)

Lightly wash then soak a two inch by two inch strip of dried wakame or kombu until soft. Cut in thin strips and place in cooking water in soup pot. Place sliced onions and carrots in soup pot and bring to boil. Immediately reduce flame to low, cover, and let simmer until onions and carrots are soft. Place three teaspoons of miso in a small bowl (or suribachi if you have one) add some soup broth and puree with a spoon, fork, or pestle until dissolved and creamy. Add this to the rest of the soup and vegetable broth and gently stir. Let simmer for two minutes and then serve. Garnish with fresh scallions, flame roasted dulse or nori, or fresh cut parsley.

If and when you reheat your miso soup for the next meal or the next day, make sure that you heat it up slowly and that you do not let the water bubble or boil! When using miso soup for medicinal purposes, never overheat and never bring to a boil or this will destroy the beneficial bacteria and enzymes. Miso soup is excellent first thing in the morning and before any whole foods meal. However do not use miso before any fresh juices. Keep these foods separated as meals or snacks or most likely they will produce gas.

Leftover miso soup can be refrigerated and used for up to three days, after that it should be discarded and a fresh batch made. Try to make only enough for two or three days at a time. The miso package or container can be stored in the refrigerator. Keep sealed.

Whole Grain Porridge - (best used for breakfast)

Ingredients and Directions

Wash and rinse thoroughly (at least 3 times) one cup of short grain organic quality brown rice (or whole oats or whole barley). I prefer the Lundberg Brothers Organic California Brown Rice, which is available at most health food stores and whole food grocery stores. In a stainless steel pressure cooker, or a stainless steel pot, add the one cup of washed and rinsed rice and 3 cups of purified tap-water (or spring water) and a pinch of organic sea salt. Add a quarter teaspoon of sea salt per one cup of rice. Use the same Celtic Sea Salt as in the watercure recipe. Stir the rice and let it settle so that the rice is evenly distributed around the bottom of the cooking pot. Bring to a boil, then set the pot on a stainless steel flame diffuser and put on a very low flame, to simmer. Simmer for at least one full hour. The longer and slower this cooks, the better the end result will be. Cook the rice (or oats or barley) until all visible water in the pot is gone. Do not stir the rice while cooking. If you are using a pressure cooker, you will just have to time it. Don't open your pressure cooker while it is hissing or making any sound whatsoever!

Everyone's stove is slightly different, so you must experiment with the amount of water and the amount of time you cook your whole grains. The goal is to achieve a soft but thick, rich and creamy consistency. Each grain of rice (or oats or barley) will have expanded fully, and the skin or shell of each grain will have ruptured. This breaking of the skin of the grain is what releases a starchy material which makes for the cream-like consistency. The end result should not be watery, not soup-like, but soft, firm, thick, and moist and somewhat sticky. It's very important for the success of your program that you learn to prepare your whole grain porridge correctly. Most of my clients are delighted to discover this recipe and report how delicious it is and how filling and satisfying too. If you get frustrated, locate a whole foods cooking instructor in your area and take some cooking classes right away.

Hipppocrates, the father of western medicine used barley porridge as a primary remedy. He would recommend hot baths or steam to induce sweating, and restrict his patient's food intake for 7 to 14 days to a simple plan of barley porridge and water. No matter what the ailment or complaint, his patients recovered quickly. This recipe for whole grain porridge is the ideal breakfast food for all ages, children, teenagers, young adults, mid-life adults and seniors. It is especially helpful on cold winter mornings. During the summer months it can be allowed to cool down to room temperature and eaten this way, but it should never been eaten cold, as in right out of the refrigerator. You can also make a fabulous rice pudding from this basic recipe by adding some raisins, cream and a little maple syrup. But save this indulgence for Phase Two of your program.

The complex carbohydrates in this whole grain porridge recipe break down very differently in the digestive system than any processed grain product you have used in the past (bread, muffins, bagels, pancakes, flaked cereals, pasta, granola, grits, oatmeal). The complex carbohydrates in whole grain porridge take longer to break down and digest and so its sugars are released more slowly over a longer period of time. This means that you will have more energy for longer periods of time after you eat it; certainly more than any other breakfast cereal or processed cereal based breakfast food you have had in the past.

During the first few weeks of Phase One of your Intestinal Regeneration Program, (in all cases of severe inflammatory bowel but not other cases) I don't want you to eat or drink anything else at your breakfast meal. Just a cup or two of cooked whole grain porridge according to the recipe above, and your warm salted drinking water according to the directions of the watercure recipe. (You can have a small bowl of miso soup before the porridge if you want.) Do not add anything to your cooked whole grain porridge. Eat it plain. This will not last forever. This is done to accelerate your intestinal healing. The food you eat during Phase One needs to be simple, organic quality whole food that is easy to digest. I have seen and heard and tried and read about every other combination of things possible. This is what has worked best for the greatest number of people over the greatest period of time. Again, this will not last forever.

You do not have to cook your porridge fresh every single day. It is absolutely not necessary. When you prepare it, cook enough to last three or four days. This way you will only need to prepare your breakfast porridge two times a week. Store your leftover porridge in your normal leftover containers. You can store it in the refrigerator. Do not use the microwave to reheat your porridge. Simply put the amount of cooked porridge you are going to consume for breakfast in a saucepan or cooking pot, and add a little water. Heat over a gentle flame. It only takes a few minutes to heat up your leftover porridge each morning.

Pressure Cooked Rice - (use for lunch or dinner)

Ingredients and Directions

Use 3 to 4 cups of spring water or purified water and 2 cups of short grain organic brown rice. Wash and rinse the rice at least 3 times, then soak the rice for 3 to 5 hours before cooking. Place the soaked brown rice and the soaking water in a pressure cooker. Add a pinch of sea salt or a ½ to ¾ inch piece of kombu in the soaking water. Secure the lid of the pressure cooker. Bring the rice up to pressure then reduce the flame to low. Put a stainless steel flame diffuser under the pressure cooker. This will prevent the bottom layer of rice from burning and sticking. Cook for about 50 minutes. Stoves vary so you will have to make adjustments. Pressure cooked rice with the above rice to water ratios creates a very different result than the recipe recommended for breakfast porridge. Pressure cooked rice will be drier, nuttier, heartier and much less wet and moist than the breakfast rice. It should be moist and all grains should be cooked thoroughly, that is puffed out to their fullest, to the point of rupturing the outer hull of the grain. Get cooking instructions or watch a cooking video demonstration if you have any questions. Once the 50 minutes cooking time is up, turn off the flame and remove the pot from the heat source. Move to a cold burner until the pressure comes down and the hissing has stopped. Once the pressure is down completely you can remove the lid of the pot. Remove the rice from the pot and place in a wooden bowel for serving. You can leave any leftover rice in the wooden bowl on the counter all day and reheat later. You can cover the leftover rice with a Japanese wooden mat used for making sushi or nori-maki or cover it with a towel.

You can easily create endless variations of tastes and textures by combining small amounts of other grains and beans in with your pressure cooked rice. Try these combinations at first, and then please feel free to create your own variations. Try 70–80% brown rice with 30–20% barley, millet, wheat, corn, or oats. These are all whole grain to whole grain combinations. Try 80–90% brown rice with 10–20% azuki beans, kidney beans, or black soybeans. These variations are for Phases Two and Three. During Phase One keep all recipes as simple and basic as possible.

Boiled Rice - (use for lunch or dinner)

Ingredients and Directions

Use a heavy pot (stainless steel, ceramic, or cast iron), with a tight fitting lid and 2 cups of spring or purified water to 1 cup of rice (or other grain) as your basic proportion. Please make sure you wash and rinse the grain at least 3 separate times and discard the rinse/wash water completely before cooking. Add a pinch of sea salt to the cooking water or a small piece of kombu or wakame seaweed (½ to ¾ inch long). Bring the water to a boil and then immediately turn the flame down low. Put the pot on a flame diffuser and simmer for about an hour or until all the water is gone.

You can easily create endless variations of tastes and textures by combining small amounts of other grains and beans in with your boiled rice. Try these combinations at first, and then please feel free to create your own variations. Try 70–80% brown rice with 30–20% barley, millet, wheat, corn, or oats. These are all whole grain to whole grain combinations. Try 80–90% brown rice with 10–20% azuki beans, kidney beans, or black soybeans. These variations are for Phases Two and Three. During Phase One keep all recipes as simple and basic as possible.

Creamed Rice

Ingredients

12 cups water
2 cups presoaked rice
pinch of sea salt or
1 inch piece of kombu

Directions

In a pressure cooker combine the water and rice. Bring to a boil over a high flame, skim off the foam, then reduce the flame, add salt and cover. Bring to pressure, then lower the flame, and cook for 30 minutes. Use a stainless steel flame diffuser under the pressure cooker while cooking. Remove from the flame and let sit until pressure comes down naturally. While still hot, process rice in a food mill, creating a creamy (milky) consistency. You still have to chew this very well but putting it through the food mill will aid in digestion.

Steamed Vegetables with Kombu
(Nishime: na-she-may)

This is a traditional Japanese recipe that is great for all digestive problems. I learned this from my friend and colleague Virginia Harper who healed herself from Crohn's Disease.

Ingredients and Directions

Use a heavy pot with a lid. Soak a ½ inch to 1 inch piece of kombu until soft and cut into ½ inch pieces. Place kombu in bottom of pot and cover with spring water. Add vegetables (see suggestions below). The vegetables should be cut into 2 inch chunks except burdock and lotus root, which should be cut smaller. Sprinkle a pinch of sea salt or shoyu over the vegetables. Cover and place on a high flame until there is a strong steam. Lower flame and cook peacefully for 20 to 30 minutes. If water evaporates during cooking, add more water to the bottom of the pot. When each vegetable has become soft and edible, add a few more drops of shoyu and mix the vegetables. Replace cover and cook over a low flame for 2 to 5 minutes. Remove cover and turn off flame. Let the vegetables sit for about 2 minutes.

Try these vegetable combinations

- onion and kombu
- onion, cabbage, carrot, squash, and kombu
- leek, carrot, and kombu
- daikon or turnip, parsnip, and kombu
- daikon, lotus root, and kombu
- carrot, cabbage, burdock, and kombu
- daikon or turnip, shiitake mushroom, and kombu

Tamari Tea

This is my favorite *emergency medicine* for stomach or intestinal gas, bloating, pain, cramping, and nausea.

One day in a restaurant, our waitress came to the table looking mighty grim-faced. "I know that expression," I said to myself, "She's in pain. She has gas!" I said to her; "Look, this is none of my business but can I ask you a question?" She nodded her head. "Are you in pain?" I asked. "Oh my God!" she replied, "I'm having the worst gas I've ever had!" Here's what I told her to do. "Go into the kitchen and grab a cup of hot water like you would if you are serving tea; just don't add any tea bags. Then go to the chef and ask for a teacup half-filled with soy sauce. Put a teaspoon of the soy sauce in the hot water and drink it down. Wait five minutes. If the pain doesn't go away in five minutes, drink another cup. Within ten minutes she came back to our table with a big smile on her face: "Oh my God!" she said, "Thank you so much! That's amazing! I have absolutely no more pain!"

Isn't it amazing how our body responds to the simplest of natural remedies?

It's best to always have on hand some organic quality *tamari*. Tamari is traditionally crafted Japanese soy sauce. It is very salty. It will neutralize an over-acid condition in the stomach and duodenum within minutes. Always use purified water whenever possible. Bring the water to a boil, and then let it cool down to somewhere between 100 and 125 degrees. Add 1 to 3 teaspoons of *tamari* per one half cup of water, stir and sip, or drink it down all at once. As you try this out a few times you will be able to determine the best way to use this recipe to create the desired result: no gas, no bloating, no stomach or intestinal pain!

This recipe/remedy can be used for emergencies and to prevent problems too. If you come to the end of the day, and feel like you over-indulged in sweets, might be feeling a bit hyper, or sugared, or stressed, make a cup of tamari tea (or two) and start drinking about an hour before bedtime. This will quiet an over acid stomach and intestine and make it easier to calm down, relax, and get a good night's sleep. Whenever you feel nauseous (including morning sickness in pregnant women), make some *tamari tea* and sip it throughout the day or as needed to relieve nausea.

Umeboshi Remedies

I learned these recipes from Dr. Marc Van Cauwenberghe in classes at the Kushi Institute in Brookline, Massachusetts in 1979 and from his book: *Macrobiotic Home Remedies*.

Background and Perspective

Pronounced, uma-bow-shee. The word is composed of two Japanese words; ume (oomay) which means plum, and boshi (bowshee) which can mean *dried or pickled*. Umeboshi is a Japanese pickled plum with outstanding medicinal properties especially helpful to people with stomach and intestinal problems.

Plums, sea salt and shiso leaves (beefsteak leaves) are all placed in a barrel, sealed, and left to ferment for at least six months or longer. When ready to eat, umeboshi plums are extremely salty to the taste and exert a powerful alkalinizing effect. Traditionally the umeboshi plum has been recommended in cases of food poisoning, water contamination, diarrhea or constipation, troubles in the stomach (too much or too little acid secretion), motion sickness, headache, and indigestion. Eating a small amount of umeboshi will neutralize excess stomach acid quickly and easily.

In the early 1950s Dr. Kyo Sato at Hirosaki University succeeded in extracting an antibiotic substance from umeboshi. He could destroy dysentery germs as well as staphylococcus. In 1968 a component was isolated from umeboshi which exerted germicidal effects against tuberculosis bacteria. Umeboshi supplies biochemical substances that secure a proper breakdown of excess acids in the blood and tissues. This helps prevent fatigue. Umeboshi contains anti-oxidant properties which are helpful in the battle against toxins and free-radicals and can therefore slow the aging process caused by oxidation. Umeboshi helps the organs responsible for detoxification and cleansing. Umeboshi helps to rejuvenate the body and increase vitality. (Marc Van Cauwenberghe, MD, *Macrobiotic Home Remedies* [Tokyo: Japan Publications, 1986], 46)

How to Use Umeboshi

You can eat a whole umeboshi plum right out of the jar, or soak it in some hot water or bancha tea and then eat it. Usually one a day is enough. Remember to use umeboshi in situations where you know there is over-acidity of the stomach; when you have stomach or intestinal problems; when there is fatigue; and after consuming too much alcohol or sugar. Some good recipes follow:

Ume-Sho-Ban (drink)

Crush the meat of one umeboshi plum in a suribachi or cup or bowl. Add ½ teaspoon of tamari soy sauce to it. Add ½ to 1 cup of hot bancha tea (or kukicha tea). You may also add several drops of fresh ginger root juice (optional). Stir well and drink slowly. This preparation is not suitable for babies or children. This drink is helpful for adults in the case of headache from too much alcohol. It is good for any indigestion, stomach aches, nausea, fatigue, anemia, weak blood, and weak circulation.

Ume-Sho-Kuzu (drink)

Dissolve a tablespoon of dried kuzu powder with two tablespoons of cold water (add the water a little at a time). Crush the meat of one umeboshi plum and add to the kuzu mix. Add 1½ to 2 cups of water to these ingredients and bring to a boil. Keep stirring the preparation slowly and gently until it becomes more or less transparent and thick. Add 1 to 3 teaspoons of tamari soy sauce. Mix and serve immediately. (Optional: add 5 to 6 drops of freshly grated ginger juice.) Use this preparation especially for stomach and intestinal problems, especially in the case of diarrhea. Consume 1 cup at a time, 2 to 3 times a day until the diarrhea has stopped.

Digestive Balance Tea

Ingredients

1/2 umeboshi plum
1/4 cup purified water
1 teaspoon kuzu powder
1/2 cup steeped kukicha (bancha) twig tea
1/2 teaspoon soy sauce
3-5 drops of ginger juice

Directions

Cut umeboshi plum into small pieces. Add the umeboshi pieces and dissolved kuzu to cool bancha tea (also called kukicha tea) and bring to a low rolling boil. This is very important since kuzu requires a boiling temperature in order to thicken. Add kuzu to water and dissolve completely. Add to low heat and stir until the cloudy kuzu turns translucent and becomes slightly thickened. Add soy sauce and ginger juice to the tea and mix ingredients together. Let cook a few more minutes. It is now ready to drink hot. This recipe is also from Virginia Harper.

Rice Balls with Umeboshi

Ingredients

- 1 cup (or more) of cooked brown rice
- 1 sheet of toasted nori sea vegetable
- 1 umeboshi plum (or some umeboshi paste)

Directions

Roast a thin sheet of nori by holding the shiny side over an open burner at a low setting about 10–12 inches from the flame. Rotate for 3–5 seconds (or longer) until the color changes from black to green. Some people prefer heating up a stainless steel flame diffuser and placing the sheet of nori on that for a few seconds to get the same result. Fold the roasted sheet of nori in half and tear it into two equal pieces. Fold these pieces in half and tear again. You should have four pieces that are about three inches on each side. Add a pinch of sea salt to a dish of water and wet your hands. Form a handful of rice into a solid ball. It can be any size you like. I usually make these to be about the size of a tennis ball. Press a hole into the rice ball with a finger and insert some umeboshi paste or a piece of an umeboshi plum inside the middle of the rice ball. Close up the hole with some rice or just re-form the ball to cover up the hole. Cover rice ball with the strips of nori, one piece at a time, until they stick. Wet your hands as needed to prevent the rice and nori from sticking to your hands, but you want the nori to stick to the rice ball.

Rice balls make for tasty, nutritious, convenient lunches or snacks because they can be eaten without utensils. Great for hiking, biking, and traveling. They will stay fresh for three or four days. Keep them in a zip-loc baggie or a small cooler. Instead of nori sheets, you can try crushed dry roasted sesame seeds (gomasio), dried wakame sheets, or green leafy vegetable leaves like kale or collard greens. Rice balls are easy to digest (as long as you chew thoroughly and slowly) and are great to calm down any digestive system problems.

I first learned this recipe from Carolyn Heidenry at our Macrobiotic Study House in Brookline, Massachusetts in 1979.

Steamed Greens

Ingredients

Enjoy steamed greens often as a delicious, nutritious, and comforting side dish to any meal; breakfast, lunch and dinner. Fresh organic greens are your best sources of minerals, especially calcium and the phytonutrient or pigment, chlorophyll; which strengthens and purifies our blood. Select any bunch or two or three of organic quality fresh greens: collards, kale, mustard greens, bok-choy, chinese cabbage, etc. Cut greens into diagonal slices or any size and shape of your liking.

Directions

Place cut greens in a stainless steel steamer tray or basket and set in place in your cooking pot. Add water to come to the bottom of the steamer tray. Bring water to a boil and cook covered until done, about 8 to 10 minutes usually. Don't overcook. Steamed greens turn a bright green when they are perfectly cooked. Learn to identify this color and match it with the proper texture of the cooked greens. The greens should not be tough to chew but they should also not be overcooked and mushy. If you overcook them, the color will not be bright green but faded green, moving towards yellowish green. Feel free to add a dash or two of tamari soy sauce as the greens are cooking. Save the steaming water for use as a soup base or to enjoy as a tasty, mineral-rich beverage in place of tea. You can also cook greens uncovered if you prefer.

Boiled Salad

This is an excellent dish for helping all digestive system problems. Traditionally, boiled salad always combined root, round and leafy green vegetables in a simple mix. Boiled or blanched vegetables should be bright and crispy, but not raw. You will know when the vegetables are ready when the color intensifies and turns brighter. Boil each vegetable separately but you can use the same water. Usually blanched vegetables for use in this boiled salad recipe are cooked for only a minute or less. Cook the mildest tasting vegetables first so that each one retains its distinctive flavor, color, and taste. Change the selection and combination of vegetables everyday. Make this dish fresh every day and always consume the vegetables within 24 hours of making. You can serve this boiled salad with or without a salad dressing. When you serve the vegetables try layering them all in a serving bowl with the heaviest vegetables on the bottom and the lightest on top.

Ingredients-Variations-Combinations

Kale, carrot, red radish, yellow onion

Red onion, chinese cabbage, daikon root

White or red cabbage, watercress, celery

Broccoli, cauliflower, carrot

Feel free to come up with your own combinations.

Directions

Select the vegetables you are going to use today from the list above or from any other combination of your own choosing. Cut, chop and slice each vegetable to your preference and set aside. Place two or three inches of spring or purified water in the bottom of a deep cooking pot. Add a pinch of sea salt. Bring to a boil. Using the kale, carrot, red radish, and yellow onion combination from above we would drop one cup of sliced yellow onion into the water for about a minute or longer and set aside. Next, drop in the kale (about 2 cups) for about a minute, then set aside. Next add one cup of sliced carrots and then one cup of sliced red radish. Cook each vegetable separately and set aside until everything is done. Then combine all vegetables in your serving bowl or dish with the heaviest vegetables on the bottom and the lightest ones on top.

Dressing Suggestions

Take one umeboshi plum or a teaspoon of umeboshi paste and add this to a ½ cup of water or use the stock from the cooking water and puree in a suribachi or small bowl. Sprinkle this on top of the layered vegetables in the serving dish or on your own individual plate. Lightly sprinkle tamari soy sauce (shoyu) over the vegetables to taste. Dilute a small amount, perhaps ½ teaspoon of barley miso with a small amount of warm water or stock from the cooking water and add a few drops of brown rice vinegar. Make a gentle mixture of a small amount of extra virgin olive oil with brown rice vinegar or balsamic vinegar and sprinkle this on the cooked vegetables.

Squash and Beans

Ingredients

Please feel free to use any combination of squashes, though winter squashes like buttercup, butternut, and hubbard are best. Please try different bean combinations too: azuki beans, kidney beans, lentils, chickpeas. You can also create variety by using onions, carrots, or parsnips instead of squash. Always use kombu or wakame seaweed when you make this to aid in digestion. The ideal proportions for this dish will approximate the following: 70% squashes or root vegetables, 25% lentils or beans, 5% kombu or wakame.

Directions

Wash and rinse the lentils or beans and then let them soak in 3 or 4 cups of water for about 5 hours. Add a 2 inch by 2 inch size piece of dried kombu to the soaking water. Remove the kombu after the 5 hour soaking and slice into thin pieces. Typically beans are cooked in a ratio of 3 cups of water to 1 cup of beans, so keep this in mind as you go forward with this recipe. You may need more water than this but probably not less. Discard the soaking water and fill the pot with pre-soaked beans with 3 or 4 cups of fresh spring water or purified water. Add the sliced kombu. Add two or three cups of chopped squash (or other vegetables of your choosing). Add more water if necessary until the water level reaches the top of the vegetable-bean mix level. Put the lid on the pot, bring to a boil then cook over a low flame for about an hour or until the beans become soft. Add more water if necessary as you cook. When the beans are soft, turn off the heat and let things sit and settle a bit before serving.

Barley with Winter Vegetables

Ingredients

- 2 inch pieces of kombu
- 2 cups whole barley, rinsed and soaked for 8 hours
- 6 cups of spring or filtered water
- Sea salt (pinch or two)
- 1 onion, chopped
- 1/2 cup of 1/2 inch cubes of rutabaga
- 1/2 cup of 1/2 inch cubes of turnip
- 1/2 cup of 1/2 inch cubes of carrots
- 1/2 cup of thinly sliced, fresh burdock root
- 2 stalks of celery, thinly sliced
- 2 or 3 dried shitake mushrooms, soaked and thinly sliced (optional)

Directions

Place kombu in a heavy pot and add barley and water. Cover and bring to a boil over medium heat. Reduce heat to low, add salt, and cook for 40 minutes. Add the vegetables, layering on top of the barley in the order listed. Re-cover the pot and cook another 40–45 minutes until the barley is creamy and vegetables are soft. Transfer to a serving bowl and serve hot. Makes 5 to 6 servings. Many thanks to Christina Pirello, for this recipe from her book *Cooking the Whole Foods Way* (NewYork: Penguin Putnam, 1997), 89.

Burdock Root and Hijiki (or Arame)

Cooked fresh burdock root is particularly beneficial in winter time. It is has a tendency to promote internal heat. It is very warming on cold winter days. It helps to keep heat inside the body. It also purifies the blood and promotes better circulation.

Ingredients

- 1 cup or one handful of hijiki or arame (either one is fine)
- 1 cup fresh burdock root, cut into small thin slices
- 1 large onion and 1 large carrot
- Water
- Tamari to taste

Directions

Wash and rinse hijiki or arame and set aside. Wash and rinse burdock root to remove all dirt/soil. Cut the burdock root on the diagonal in thin slices, about one quarter inch thick. Set aside. Cut carrots into slices on the diagonal too, but thicker. In a large cast iron skillet or stainless steel frying pan, sauté one large onion or two small onions. You can use a little sesame oil or canola oil. When the onions become translucent, turn the heat down all the way to a simmer. Add the sliced carrots and the sliced burdock. Add the hijiki or arame. Add enough water to almost cover the vegetables and seaweed. Add a pinch or two of sea salt. Bring to a boil, cover and then reduce the flame to a simmer again. Simmer until vegetables are done. The burdock will be chewy but when done you will easily bite through it. It will taste earthy. Season with tamari to taste and then simmer another 15–20 minutes. This will guarantee proper cooking of the burdock. Remove the cover from pan and cook away the excess liquid. Season with tamari to taste and serve.

Japanese Noodle Soup with Tofu

Ingredients

   4 cups of spring or filtered water
   1 2 inch long piece of kombu
   1 dried shitake mushroom (optional)
   1 cup of ¼ inch cut cubes of tofu
   4 to 6 ounces of udon or soba noodles, cooked al dente, drained and rinsed.
   1 or 2 green onions or scallions cut into thin diagonal slices
   1/2 sheet of nori, shredded (optional)

Directions

Bring water to a boil in a soup pot. Add kombu and shitake mushroom, cover, and simmer for ten minutes. Remove kombu and mushroom and season lightly with tamari soy sauce. You have just made a traditional Japanese broth called dashi, which is used as a soup base or dipping sauce in many recipes. Stir in tofu cubes. Simmer another ten minutes. Divide the precooked noodles among individual soup bowls and ladle soup over noodles. Serve garnished with sliced scallions and shredded nori. You can also thinly slice the cooked kombu and shitake mushroom and add back to the broth before ladling over the noodles. Makes four servings. This recipe is from Christina Pirello.

Black Bean Soup

Ingredients

1 cup dried black turtle beans, soaked overnight
1 quart water
1 large onion
3 medium cloves of garlic
1 tablespoon extra-virgin olive oil
1 tomato
1/4 teaspoon dried oregano
1/2 teaspoon ground cumin
2 teaspoons chili powder
1 bay leaf
2 tablespoons of mirin (sweet rice wine) or 1 tablespoon of dry sherry
1½ tablespoons brown rice vinegar
sea salt and freshly ground black pepper to taste
1/4 cup chopped whole scallions for garnish just before serving

Directions

Drain the beans and place them in a 6-quart soup pot with water. Bring to a boil, skimming the foam that rises to the surface until it almost ceases to form, then reduce heat, cover and cook for 45 minutes. While the beans are cooking, chop the onion fine and mince the garlic. In a medium skillet, heat the oil and sauté the onion and garlic over medium heat for 4 or 5 minutes. While onion and garlic are sautéing, drop the tomato into the bean pot for 30 seconds; remove using a slotted spoon. Peel. Cut in half crosswise and squeeze out the seeds. Chop coarsely and add to the skillet, along with the oregano, cumin and chili powder. Cook, stirring for 2 or 3 minutes. Scrape the contents of the skillet into the soup pot. Add the bay leaf. Cover the pot and simmer for 1 more hour.

Add the mirin or sherry, vinegar, and salt and pepper and continue to simmer for another 30 minutes. If you wish, puree 2 to 3 cups of soup in a blender or food processor to create a thicker, smoother texture. Remove the bay leaf. Ladle into soup bowls and serve, garnished with chopped scallions.

Many thanks to Annemarie Colbin for this recipe from her book *The Natural Gourmet*. Do not use this recipe in Phase One. Save it for Phase Two and beyond.

Section 3 - Optimizing Results

Recipe for Rice Pudding

Depending on the severity of your symptoms, you will need to save this recipe until you have restored some measure of normal functioning. Once that is achieved you should be able to enjoy this recipe and many others on a regular basis.

Ingredients

3 1/2 cups of cooked brown rice (short grain, medium or long grain rice)
1 1/2 cups of apple juice (or half water and half juice)
1/4 teaspoon of sea salt
1/3 to 1/2 cup of water
1/4 teaspoon of cinnamon
1/2 cup of almonds
3/4 cup of water
3/4 of a tablespoon of tahini

Directions

Boil almonds in three quarters cup of water with three quarters of a tablespoon of tahini. Puree in a blender. Place all ingredients in a pressure-cooker and cook for 40–45 minutes. Allow pressure to come down. Place ingredients in a baking dish or covered casserole dish and bake at 350 degrees for 45 minutes to an hour. Remove cover and brown top.

This recipe is from the book *Macrobiotic Cooking for Everyone* by Wendy Esko. (You do not have to use a pressure cooker.)

The Conscious Breathing Exercise

When it comes to the fundamentals of nutrition and health, it doesn't get any more fundamental than oxygen. Although I have not emphasized this at all throughout the text so far, I should have. Oxygen is a vital nutrient, perhaps the most vital of all. We can go without food and water for days at a time. We can go without oxygen, in the form of normal breathing, for only a few minutes. The air we breath is a most precious and vital nutrient. Most people do not breathe correctly and therefore are unintentionally insulting the normal oxygenation of blood, lymph, organs, and cells on a continual basis. The foundation of every traditional medical and meditation tradition is proper breathing. Proper breathing is one of the first complementary habits I learned in the earliest days of my healing journey. Proper breathing is one of the most important habits we can teach ourselves and share with the people we care about the most. Here is the basic explanation I give to my clients.

Tension anywhere in the body will reduce circulation and make it difficult for normal functioning to take place. Tension in the abdomen can be partly or entirely responsible for many uncomfortable digestive system problems. We must all learn to relax. The key to relaxation is proper breathing.

This is a simple explanation of yogic breathing or abdominal breathing. Practicing this breathing exercise for only ten full breaths, two or three times a day, can be very effective in alleviating many symptoms of imbalance and disharmony. Some of these symptoms include: anger, depression, anxiety, worry, fatigue and indigestion.

Section 3 - Optimizing Results

There are many others. Proper breathing will increase oxygen flow throughout the body, help you relax and help you manage your negative stress more effectively.

Sit in a comfortable chair, or lie on the floor on your back. If you lie on the floor, make sure you have a pad or blanket to lie on. You need to be comfortable for this to work. Close your eyes, or keep them open slightly and gently focused on a point on the floor or ceiling. Focus on a point on the floor if you are sitting in a chair. Focus on a point on the ceiling if you are lying down on the floor. Notice how you are breathing normally. Notice how much time it takes for a normal breath to come in and go out. Are you breathing through your nose or through your mouth? How deep does the breath get into your body? Can you feel the breath down to the bottom of each lung? Or does it feel like your breath gets stuck somewhere half-way down your throat? Most of us, without conscious effort and attention to the contrary, are shallow breathers. Shallow breathing on a regular and continual basis can lead to tension, nervousness, anxiety and deprive our cells of the complete oxygen supply they need to function normally.

Let's begin the conscious breathing exercise right now. Go slowly. Take your time. Relax.

Let all the air out of your lungs through your mouth, and when it is all out, exaggerate your out-breath by blowing outwards a few more seconds. When you do this, you should notice a slight contraction in your upper abdomen, just below your rib cage. If you have never tried this before, you have just succeeded in your first conscious abdominal breath! The muscle just below your rib cage that acts like a bellows when we exercise it properly is called the diaphragm. Diaphragmatic or abdominal (or yogic) breathing is the most effective way to oxygenate our blood without more elaborate exercise programs. It can be done almost anywhere (as long as you don't mind other people staring at you).

Try breathing in through both nostrils this time, and as you draw in this new breath, do it as slowly and methodically as possible. Exaggerate the slowness and luxuriate in the simple act of taking in a larger than normal volume of air into your lungs. Remember to go slowly. No rush, no hurry. It will take a while to get the hang of this. Imagine the air descending to the bottom of each lung, and diffusing out of the lungs and into the rest of your body. Visualize the oxygen diffusing into your blood and from there outwards into every cell in your entire body.

Section 3 - Optimizing Results

Imagine the oxygen attracting and gathering a variety of gaseous toxins into itself and then, at the point when you can no longer comfortably keep breathing in...pause for a few seconds...then simply become aware that you have completely filled every square inch of space inside your lungs. At the point of your fullest lung capacity, yet still remaining completely relaxed and comfortable and no tension anywhere, begin to very slowly exhale through your mouth, as if you were letting the air out of a very large balloon a little bit at a time. Visualize the release of all that carbon dioxide and all those other toxins attached to it. Visualize the millions of little air sacs (alveoli), cleansed of all their impurities. Visualize that every cell in your entire body just received a better supply of oxygen and got rid of many unwanted and dangerous toxins. When your exhalation is complete, force out just a little more air, but stay comfortable.

Pause a quiet second or two before you begin a new inhalation. With the new inhalation, see if you can taste and feel the quality of the air you are breathing in as it streams in through your nostrils, some into your mouth and around your tongue, down your throat, and into your lungs. Exaggerate the inhalation and consciously pull the air into the center of your belly and fill up your entire abdomen as if it were a giant bellows or hot air balloon. Once filled, repeat the exercise as described above. Repeat this exercise a minimum of ten times and with each inhalation and exhalation, see if you notice any changes in how your body-mind responds. Do this slowly in a gentle series of ten complete breaths. Do it three times a day for a week and see if you notice any changes in your overall energy, vitality, sense of alertness and sense of calmness.

Of course, if you would like to do this longer than ten breaths, feel free. Most people who use this exercise or some variant as part of their regular habit of meditation usually suggest a time frame between twenty and forty minutes, twice daily for optimum results.

Therapeutic Abdominal Massage

According to traditional natural healing models of health, the major cause of every symptom, sickness and disease can explained away with one word: blockage. Blocked energy, blocked circulation of blood and lymph, blockages caused from tense muscles. Even thoughts and emotions that are blocked, as in unexpressed or unspoken can be part of the problem. Obviously if you are constipated you are familiar with the feeling of blockage. One of the simplest, easiest, and most effective things we can do to address the symptoms of any degree of blockage anywhere in our body is massage; gentle, focused, therapeutic touch. Here is a basic explanation for an effective abdominal massage.

You must be comfortable for this to work. It is best if you are lying down flat on your back. You can lie on your bed or on the floor. Lie on a padded mat or blanket. Make sure you are comfortable. Let's begin:

Place both of your hands, palms down on either side of your navel. Trace a circle around your navel with the index finger of your choice. This is the deepest part of your small intestine. Now start another circle just outside of the first one. Keep doing this until you come to the last three or four inches around the entire periphery of your abdomen. This will be the outline of your entire Large Intestine. This massage will focus on the Large Intestine. You can use this same technique to massage the area containing the Small Intestine as well.

Two or three finger widths in from the point of your right hip bone, the part of the hip bone that juts deepest into your abdomen, is your appendix. The appendix is on the Large Intestine side of your ileo-cecal valve. This valve marks the end of the small intestine (ileum) and the start of the large intestine (cecum). Moving in a vertical line up the right side of your body is the *ascending colon*. It makes a sharp turn underneath your right rib cage (location of your liver/gall bladder) and flows across your abdomen a good hands width or more above your navel. This is called your *transverse colon*. The transverse colon crosses the spine at the L5-S1 vertebrate. Ask any chiropractor in the world and you will discover that this is the location where most problems occur along the spine. Why? Unhealthy transverse colons. A healthy vibrant colon supports the spine. An unhealthy colon has a weakening effect on the health of the spine.

Underneath your left rib cage, the transverse colon takes another sharp turn downwards and runs south to the location of your left hip bone. The sharp turn down is called the *splenic flexure*. Underneath your left rib cage is the location of your spleen and pancreas. This section of the colon is called the descending colon. The descending colon descends to the left hip bone and turns south again to a location a few inches below the navel, making an S-like curve in the process. This is called the *Sigmoid Colon*. At last, the sigmoid colon turns into the rectum and at the bottom of the rectum is the anus.

There is a simple but highly therapeutic self-massage you can give to this entire area, with particular emphasis on the entire large intestine. This abdominal massage is helpful for all digestive system problems and will be particularly effective in cases of mild constipation. It will also help if there is mild bloating, discomfort and gas. This gentle massage will increase peristalsis and if you do it thoroughly enough it will help you to locate any potential problem areas. The entire abdominal area should be soft, pliable and flexible. As you press down on it (I will explain this in a minute), you should not feel any pain and you should not feel anything hard. If you do feel any pain or any hardness, take note of it and write it down in your journal. Give the exact location and description to your Primary Health Care Provider. It could simply be the location of what is called a fecal impaction which is basically some old hardened poop. If it doesn't soften and go away after two or three colon cleanses, then you would most likely need to get an x-ray, ultrasound, or ctscan and see what else it might be.

Make sure you are lying down on your back on the floor, or on your bed. Be comfortable. No TV or radio or loud music. You need it to be quiet. You need to listen and feel for things in your abdomen. You need to coordinate the gentle pressing down of your fingertips (explanation follows) with deep and slow abdominal breathing. Coordinate the

Section 3 - Optimizing Results

activity of this abdominal massage with the steps of the Conscious Breathing Exercise for best results. Each time you breathe out, breathe out long and slowly. Press down on your abdomen with your fingertips. Start at the twelve o'clock position. This should be right in the middle of your transverse colon. Put your two hands together into a normal prayer position. Palms touching, fingers lined up against each other. Then gently, slowly, curl your fingertips downwards until the backs of your hands and fingers are now touching. Then, at the start of your exhalation, press down firmly but gently with your (inverted) fingertips at the twelve o'clock position of your abdomen. Go down as deeply as you can, but slowly. If you feel any pain or discomfort, just ease up. Take notice, and go to the next position which is one o'clock. Go clockwise around your abdomen, one breath at a time. With each new exhalation press down on the next position: two o'clock, three o'clock, etc. Go all the way around back to twelve o'clock. Do this at least three times all the way around. You should succeed in pressing down on every square inch of your entire large intestine. You may hear gurgling. You may feel some pressure or tension or tightness. You may feel some discomfort. You should not feel any serious pain. If you feel any level of serious pain you should see your doctor right away. You may feel the presence of some bowel movement material, in the area of the sigmoid colon. Take good mental notes and when you are done, write down some notes in your journal. What did you discover?

The best time to do this abdominal massage is first thing in the morning. With practice you may find that it helps you to eliminate in the morning and become more regular. Combine this with all my other suggestions and your entire digestive system will be much happier and function better. If you have never done this before, do it once a day for at least seven days in a row. Pay attention to what you are experiencing. Take notes. Keep a journal.

Eat Light and Eat Early

There is no question that how and when and where and why we eat are all as important and often more important factors in determining our digestive system health than what we eat. Eating when stressed, overeating, eating standing up, and a lack of proper chewing are all insulting habits and will contribute to various symptoms and conditions of digestive dis-ease. However, there is one insulting habit that towers over them all: eating late at night. Our body is intimately connected and associated with the natural rhythms of the earth and none of these ancient rhythms is more influential than the rising and setting of the sun. For thousands of years (with rare exceptions throughout the year), our ancestors got up before sunrise and retired soon after sunset. There was no electricity and no television or radio to distract them. Their lives were centered on their work and most of them were farmers. This meant that they had to take advantage of the available sunlight. The main meal of the day was usually the first meal. After several hours of work, another meal was taken at mid-day. Once all the equipment, tools, and work animals were put away at the end of the day, it was already dark. Rarely was a third meal taken. And if it was, it was often light soups, bread crusts or gruel.

> Early to bed and early to rise makes a man healthy, wealthy, and wise.
> Benjamin Franklin

During the daylight hours is the optimum time for digestion. After sunset, the body wants to rest and sleep. The body never rests

Section 3 - Optimizing Results

completely of course. Internal body temperatures are maintained, blood continues to be pumped and circulated. Trillions of cells take in nutrients, produce products, and eliminate waste products. Rest is a relative term inside the human body. Recalling our each cell is a factory analogy, we can imagine that the busiest factories also never totally shut down either. Production is usually highest during the daylight hours. At night, the factory must be cleaned up and repaired, in preparation for the next day's activities. And so it is inside the human body.

Digestion of food uses up a lot of energy and resources and while digesting is going on, other important activities suffer. During rest and sleep in the overnight hours, our body wants and needs to be focused on internal cleansing and repair work at the cellular level. If this most vital and essential physiological priority of the body is constantly insulted and interfered with, by eating late at night, there will be symptoms and conditions as a result. The body tries to tell us these things often in the form of restless sleep or crazy dreams and nightmares, often in the form of early morning fatigue. Of course, like all the other habits I have talked to you about it, the easiest way to prove the validity of this one is to experiment.

Remember that when the digestive system is stressed it will convert food energy into fat. This means that the easiest way to lose weight is to not eat late at night. Late at night is a relative term. The best times to eat are between sunrise and sunset. Anything we eat after sunset will digest less well than if we ate it before sunset.

Millions of people suffer from insomnia and other restless sleep disorders. The number one cause?—indigestion from eating too late at night. I suffered from insomnia as a teenager for almost five years. When I had my first official consultation with someone skilled in the arts of Functional Nutrition I asked about the cause and cure for insomnia. I was asked if I had the habit of eating anything before going to bed. I shared that every night before going to bed I had a big bowl of ice cream with chocolate sauce and whipped cream. I was told to "experiment" and not do that for a week or two to see what would happen. I experimented. No more insomnia. This was a powerful lesson for me.

In hundreds of lectures around the country and in many telephone consultations over the years people have told me stories about their grandparent's relationship to this habit of not eating late at night. It is almost universal. Healthy people living into their eighties and nineties all shared this habit of eating less, chewing more and not eating late at night.

At one lecture in the mid 1990s in Boston, a very excited Russian woman couldn't wait to tell me about a saying she had learned as a child: *Have breakfast with yourself. Have lunch with a friend. Give supper to your enemy!* If you still have any doubt whatsoever about the power and influence of this habit on your digestive system, I have this advice for you: experiment! A word to the wise is sufficient.

Section 3 - Optimizing Results

The Habits: Daily and Weekly Checklists

Making the transition to a healthier diet and lifestyle can most effectively be achieved by understanding and then consistently practicing the most important health and nutrition fundamentals. I have attempted to explain most of them throughout the course of this book. Here is a simple checklist to help you remember the difference between the complementary habits and the insulting ones. I suggest you check this list twice daily, at the beginning and at the end of each day. If you minimize and/or completely avoid the insulting habits while practicing and optimizing the complementary habits you will succeed in gradually yet dramatically improving the quality of your health and life!

Primary habits to consider

1. Check this list each morning
2. Proper sleep last night? Any dreams? (record in your journal)
3. Proper daily hydration
4. Moderate exercise each day
5. Conscious breathing exercise
6. Therapeutic Abdominal Massage
7. Selecting better quality food
8. Selecting better quality beverages
9. Improved preparation of foods
10. Always sit down when you eat
11. Always be calm when you eat
12. Always say "grace" before and after meals

13. Always eat slowly and chew
14. Never eat to fullness; listen!
15. Do not eat and run; relax first!
16. Avoid cold foods and beverages
17. Avoid eating anything late in the day
18. Check this list before going to bed

Additional habits to consider

1. Daily superfood supplements
2. Daily green drink plus
3. Digestive enzymes before meals
4. Probiotics before meals
5. Anti-oxidant supplements daily
6. Eat fruit separate from other foods
7. 16 to 32 oz of fresh juice each day (optional)
8. Cooked, whole grain cereal daily
9. Lightly steamed vegetables daily
10. Dry roasted seeds and nuts daily
11. Small amount of cooked beans daily (optional)
12. Raw fruits and vegetables daily (raw can be optional)
13. Small portions of organic quality meat/fish when desired

Reduce and minimize these habits

1. Dairy foods in general; milk, cheese, butter
2. Beer, wine, alcohol
3. Processed foods in general
4. Baked flour products, bread, donuts, cookies, cakes, pies
5. Processed/packaged breakfast cereals
6. Deep fried foods
7. Fast food restaurant food
8. Carbonated beverages of any kind
9. Sodas and diet sodas
10. Candy bars and all other junk food snacks

Section 3 - Optimizing Results

Seek to eliminate these habits

1. Microwave oven use
2. Food additives and preservatives
3. Food colorings and dyes
4. Herbicides and pesticides
5. Anything artificial
6. Meats that contain antibiotics
7. Meats that contain growth hormones
8. Meats that contain pesticides
9. Any foods containing GMO's
10. Drinking unfiltered tap water

Additional habits to consider

1. Whole foods cooking classes
2. Backyard organic gardening
3. Join a local CSA group
4. Growing your own sprouts
5. Regular use of a juicer
6. Periodic fasting
6. Seasonal cleansing
7. Natural fiber clothing
8. Toxin free personal products
9. Toxin free workplace and home

Self-evaluation habits:

1. Colon transit time
2. Two or three bowel movements per day
3. Quality of bowel movements
4. Fecal incontinence?
5. Color of first urine of day
6. Urgency of urine flow
7. Quantity of urine flow
8. Urinary incontinence?
9. Body odor in general
10. Quality of breath
11. Skin quality

12. Skin brushing
13. Brightness in eyes
14. Whiteness of white part of eye
15. Overall aches and pains
16. Moods
17. Physical energy
18. Mental clarity
19. Memory
20. My personal vision, mission and purpose in life!
21. Am I living my life to the fullest?

Section Four
WHAT'S NEXT?

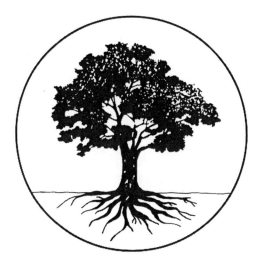

Food is the soil from which the tree of our own life is grown.

Section 4 - What's Next

About the Author

Russell Mariani is the director of client services at The Center for Functional Nutrition in South Hadley, Massachusetts. He is a Health Educator and Nutrition Counselor and has been in private practice since 1980. He has his Bachelor's degree from Rutgers University, a Masters degree in Nutrition Counseling from Norwich University, and continues acquiring ongoing education credits in the area of Digestive Wellness. Since 1980 he has helped thousands of people regain their health through dietary and lifestyle improvements through classes, seminars, retreats and personal consultations. He is passionate about teaching others how to become more proactive in their own self-care.

"My interest in natural healing and whole foods nutrition began shortly after I was mis-diagnosed with colon cancer in 1973. Within three months the doctors settled on a diagnosis of *pre-cancerous ulcerative colitis*. I was 18 years old at the time. Believing I had little time to live and no time to waste, I started on my healing quest. I sought the answers to a few questions of vital interest to me at the time: How did this happen to me? What are the *root causes* of digestive disease? What role does diet and lifestyle play in reversing the disease process and restoring one's vitality, energy, health? Just exactly *how* does health really work? The answers I found were so inspiring and helpful that I decided to dedicate the rest of my life to the continuous learning and teaching of the fundamentals of nutrition and health. And that's what I've been doing since 1980. What you will find in the pages of this book, *Healing Digestive Illness*, is a concise summary of all the things I have learned and all the things I try to teach my clients working closely

Section 4 - What's Next

together with them one-on-one over the course of several months. Please let me know how this book has helped you to heal yourself from any digestive system problem you have been suffering from and please do not hesitate to contact me directly by phone (413-536-0275) or through my website, www.healingdigestiveillness.com if you are interested in a private consultation.

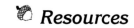

Resources

The Center for Functional Nutrition
Russell Mariani and Megan Moore, Directors
514 Amherst Road
South Hadley, MA 01075
www.healingdigestiveillness.com
413-536-0275 (consultations only)
413-536-3322 (all other inquiries)

We named the Center in 1999 before the terms Functional Nutrition and Functional Medicine became popular. Our center is a virtual center in that all of our clients are serviced via phone, email or Skype. We have clients all around the world. Although our primary focus is Digestive Wellness, we provide comprehensive wellness services that cover all other health conditions and concerns. Please let us know how we can help you to achieve your optimum health and healing goals.

Global Health Solutions
PO Box 3189
Falls Church, VA 22043
www.watercure.com
800-759-3999

Global Health Solutions publishes Dr. F. Batmanghelidji's (Dr. B.) pioneering work on the connections between *chronic unintentional dehydration* and a vast array of human diseases previously believed to be *incurable*. His first book; *Your Body's Many Cries for Water* radically changed my life and completely transformed my state of health and well-being. There is nothing easier and more profound that every person wanting to increase the quality of their life and health can do than learn the habit of proper daily hydration! Dr. B is the man who discovered the watercure, which one day may prove to be the single greatest health discovery of the twentieth century!

Multipure International
7251 Cathedral Rock Drive
Las Vegas, NV 89128
www.mutipure.com
800-622-9206

Multi-Pure makes the best point of use drinking water systems in the world, period. It is the only water purifier I have used and recommended for almost 30 years. Check out the information on their website. Most of my clients order the Aquaversa. Then call my office at 413-536-3322 when you are ready to place your order. In almost 30 years I have never had anyone return a unit or complain about performance. 100% customer satisfaction is almost unheard of with any product but that has been my experience with Multipure. I still use the same stainless steel unit I bought in 1987. It looks brand new. All I do is replace the inner cartridge or "filter" once a year. Pure drinking and cooking water for about 8 cents a gallon. Fantastic product!

The Grain & Salt Society
4 Celtic Drive
Arden, NC 29704
www.celticseasalt.com
800-867-7258

The Celtic Sea Salt from the Grain and Salt Society is the very best salt in the whole wide world. I have been using organic sea salt on my food and in my cooking water for over forty years. I have been adding the Celtic Sea Salt to my drinking water per the steps of the watercure recipe since 1997. It is not only the best quality salt in the world, it's the best tasting too. Also visit: www.selinanaturally.com

American Botanical Pharmacy
PO Box 9459
Marina del Rey, CA 90295
www.herbdoc.com
800-437-2362

The American Botanical Pharmacy is the home of Dr. Richard Schulze who is the greatest formulator of organic quality and wild harvested herbal products in the world. He is a passionate natural healing evangelist! I have used and recommended his products since I first discovered them in 1997. Without the use and benefits of his Intestinal Formulas, my Intestinal Regeneration Program would not be as effective as it is. His Intestinal Formulas are simply the best I have ever found, period. Check with Megan Moore in our office and request an updated Product List and Product Usage Guidelines pdf. 413-536-3322.

Virginia Harper
Digestive Wellness Educator
106 Seminole Drive
Franklin, TN 37069
www.youcanhealyou.com
615-646-2841

Virginia Harper is my good friend and most trusted colleague in the world of digestive wellness. She frequently conducts residential programs and retreats for direct hands-on guidance and support. She is the author of *Controlling Crohn's Disease the Natural Way* which is now in its third edition.

Libby Barnett
The Reiki Healing Connection
633 Isaac Frye Hwy
Wilton, N.H. 03086
www.reikienergy.com
603-654-2787

My friend Libby Barnett is coauthor of *Reiki Energy Medicine: Bringing Healing Touch into Home, Hospital and Hospice.* This book has sold over 70,000 copies and is printed in seven languages. It is a great introduction to Reiki, which is a gentle, hands-on form of energy healing. It includes many examples of how Reiki can be integrated with conventional healthcare to reduce stress, manage pain and promote healing. Libby has taught Reiki to over 8,000 people, including many healthcare professionals in many of the major hospitals in the northeastern United States. Check out her website for more information. www.reikienergy.com

Lotus Seed Press
12 Hayes Ave
Northampton, MA 01060
www.lotusseedpoetry.com
413-586-9923

Lotus Seed Press is the best place to find the poetry books and cds of Danny Shanahan. I have known Danny for over thirty years after first meeting him in the Open Sesame Café in Brookline, MA in 1979 while we were both writing poetry at separate tables during the mid-afternoon restaurant lull. In my humble opinion, Danny is one of the best poets of our generation and he lives and breathes the life of the Great Irish Tenors and Wandering Minstrels of his celtic bardic ancestors. He is a true wild man, with a heart of gold and a voice that can make the angels cry. Please visit his site and buy his books and cds! His books, cds and live performances are among the things in this life that nourish me best.

Robert Smyth - Design & Audio Production
29 Josephine Ave
Somerville, MA 02144-2312
smyth.rb@gmail.com
617-776-2230

If you want to produce a book, pamphlet, brochure, or CD to tell the story of what you do, Robert can help you do that. With 25 plus years experience in production and design he will lead you through the journey of publishing materials to augment your work. He founded Yellow Moon Press in 1979, to explore and revitalize the oral tradition as it pertains to storytelling, poetry and music.

Note from RM: Robert designed the first and second editions of *Healing Digestive Illness*.

Section 4 - What's Next

🌰 Sources for Organic Quality Whole Foods

Whole Foods Market
525 North Lamar
Austin, TX 78703
www.wholefoodsmarket.com
512-476-1206

Whole Foods Market is the world's largest retailer of natural and organic foods with over 340 stores throughout North America and the United Kingdom with more stores opening everywhere on a continual basis. Whole Foods Market is the future of supermarket and grocery shopping. If you have never been inside of one of these stores you are in for a big treat and a very pleasant surprise. Take advantage of all the services these stores provide. You can buy the very best cookware. You can take whole foods cooking classes. You can also locate the very best holistic health care providers in your area. Don't forget to support local agriculture!

Eden Foods
701 Tecumseh Road
Clinton, MI 49236
888-441-3336
www.edenfoods.com

Jaffe Brothers
Organic Fruits and Nuts
28560 Lilac Road
Valley Center, CA 92032
www.organicfruitsandnuts.com
760-749-1133

Gold Mine Natural Food Company
7805 Anjons Drive
San Diego, CA 92126
www.goldminenaturalfood.com
800-475-3663

Natural Lifestyle
16 Lookout Drive
Asheville, NC 28804
www.natural-lifestyle.com
800-752-2772

Miracle Exclusives
Mostly Kitchen Equipment
64 Seaview Blvd.
Port Washington, NY 11050
www.miracleexclusives.com
800-645-6360

Community Supported Agriculture (CSA) is an excellent way for the food buying public to create a win-win relationship with a local organic farm and receive a weekly basket of the very best local produce during the growing season. For more information please go to www.localharvest.com

🌰 Great Cookbooks, DVD's, & Cooking Instructors

Christina Pirello, *Cooking The Whole Foods Way*, (and many other books). Christina became a vegetarian at the age of fourteen. In 1983, after being diagnosed with terminal leukemia, she decided to forego conventional medical treatments and turned to nutrition and whole foods cooking, to heal herself. For the past 30 years Christina has been teaching whole foods cooking classes, catering and lecturing nationwide. Today she can be seen regularly on her award winning PBS television program, *Christina Cooks!* For some of the most enlightening and entertaining books and dvd's on the subject go to: www.christinacooks.com

Annemarie Colbin, Ph.D. Dr. Colbin is one of the pioneers of the whole foods movement and her 1984 classic, *Food and Healing* still remains one of the pivotal statements about the connections between diet and health ever written. She started the *Natural Gourmet Cookery School* in New York City and has been responsible for the education and training of hundreds of the world' most skilled natural food chefs. This school is now called, *The Natural Gourmet Institute for Food and Health*. 48 West 21st Street, 2nd floor (between 5th and 6th Avenues) New York, New York, 10010. 212-645-5170. For more information about Dr. Colbin's books, dvds, upcoming lectures, appearances, etc. please visit two websites: www.foodandhealing.com and www.naturalgourmetschool.com

Meredith McCarty NE, is the author of three cookbooks including the international award winning, *Sweet and Natural*. She is an associate of Physicians Committee for Responsible Medicine and has worked in educational programs with Drs. Benjamin Spock, Dean Ornish, John McDougall and Neal Barnard. She is former associate editor of *East West/Natural Health* magazine and the co-director of the East West Center for Natural Health Education for almost 30 years. Meredith studied macrobiotics with Michio and Aveline Kushi and with Herman and Cornelia Aihara in the 1970's. She has a Senior Certificate in the Art of Cooking from the Kushi Foundation, and received Nutrition Educator certification from Bauman College. For more information on her cooking classes, talks and membership in her Health E-Club, visit Meredith's website: www.healingcuisine.come

Linda (Wemhoff) Michael's *Cooking for Health and Vitality* is a favorite for my clients. The instructional dvd is designed for beginners but serves as a great review of important fundamentals for more experienced whole foods enthusiasts as well. Seasonal menu plans, recipes, recipes for delicious meals and a link to her youtube videos can be found at www.macrobioticcooking.com

Residential Programs

Sometimes the very best thing to do is to find a residential healing facility that is completely devoted to teaching you all the fundamentals of how to select, prepare and then consciously consume your foods. Here are the best of the best!

The Ki of Life Learning Center
106 Seminole Drive
Franklin, TN 37069
www.youcanhealyou.com
615-646-2841

Virginia (Ginny) Harper healed herself from a life-threatening condition that included Crohn's Disease (and many other serious medical complications) over 30 years ago. She wrote a book about her amazing healing journey, *Controlling Crohn's Disease The Natural Way*, and has been teaching others how to heal themselves ever since. Ginny is one of my most trusted colleagues and one of the world's great experts about healing digestive disorders through proper diet and lifestyle changes.

Kripalu Center for Yoga and Health
PO Box 793
West Street, route 183
Lenox, MA 01240
www.kripalu.org
866-200-5203 (toll free)
413-448-3152 (international and local)

The Kushi Institute
198 Leland Road
Beckett, MA 01223
www.kushiinstitute.org
programs@kushiinstitute.org
800-975-8744 (toll free)
413-623-5741 (international and local)

The Institute for Integrative Nutrition
120 West 41st Street second floor
New York, NY 10036
www.integrativenutrition.com
212-730-5433 (international and local)
877-730-5444 (toll free)

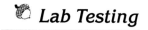

Lab Testing

Genova Diagnostics
63 Zillicoa Street
Asheville, NC 28806
www.gdx.net
800-522-4762 (toll free)
828-253-0621 (international and local)

Genova Diagnostics is a global leader in functional laboratory testing, pioneering innovative new approaches to Functional and Personalized Medicine.

Select Bibliography

Abrams, K. (1996). *Algae to the Rescue.* Studio City, CA: Logan House Publications.

Aihara, H. (1980). *Acid and Alkaline.* Oroville, CA: George Ohsawa Foundation.

Airola, P. (1971). *Are You Confused?* Phoenix, AZ: Health Plus Publishers.

American Cancer Society. (2003). *Cancer Facts & Figures.* Atlanta: GA.

Anderson, J. (1999). *How problems with digestion can cause illness anywhere in the body.* In Nichols, T. & Faass, N., (Ed.). *Optimal Digestion: New Strategies for Achieving Digestive Health.* (pp. 125-135). New York: Avon Books.

Anderson, R. (1992). *Cleanse and Purify Thyself.* Tucson, AZ: Arise & Shine Inc.

Balch, P. (2000). *Prescription for Nutritional Healing.* New York: Avery Books.

Ballantine, R. (1986). *Diet and Nutrition: A Holistic Approach.* Honesdale, PA: The Himalayan International Institute.

Batmanghelidj, F. (1996). *Your Body's Many Cries for Water.* Falls Church, VA: Global Health Solutions.

Batmanghelidj, F. (2000). *ABC of Asthma, Allergies & Lupus.* Falls Church, VA: Global Health Solutions.

Batmanghelidj, F. (2004). *Obesity, Cancer, Depression,* Falls Church, VA: Global Health Solutions.

Becker, W. (2000). *The World of the Cell.* San Francisco: Addison Wesley Longman.

Bennett, C. (2000). *Black & White Of An Empty Harvest.* Durango: Spirit Symbols.

Bly, R. (1973). *Sleepers Joining Hands.* New York: Harper & Row.

Bly, R. (1975). *The Morning Glory: Prose Poems.* New York: Harper & Row.

Bly, R. (1976). *The Kabir Book.* Boston: Beacon Press

Bly, R. (1980). *News Of The Universe.* Editor: San Francisco: Sierra Club Books.

Bly, R. (1981). *I Am Too Alone In The World.* New York: Silver Hands Press.

Bly, R. (1986). *A Little Book On The Human Shadow.* Memphis: Racoon Books.

Bly, R. (1990). *Iron John.* New York: Addison-Wesley Publishing Company.

Bly, R. (1993). *The Rag And Bone Shop Of The Heart.* New York: Harper Collins.

With Michael Meade and James Hillman as co-editors.

Bly, R. (1996). *The Sibling Society.* New York: Addison-Wesley Publishing.

Boyle, T. (1993). *The Road to Wellville.* New York: Viking Press.

Brody, D. (1996). *The Science Class You Wish You Had.* New York: The Berkeley Publishing Group.

Bruno, J. (2001). *Edible Microalgae: A Review of the Health Research.* Pacifica, CA: The Center for Nutritional Psychology Press.

Campbell, J. (1949). *The Hero With A Thousand Faces.* Princeton: Princeton University Press.

Campbell, J. (1959). *The Masks Of God.* New York: Penguin Books.

Campbell, J. (1988). *Historical Atlas Of World Mythology.* New York: Harper & Row.

Campbell, C.T. (2006). *The China Study.* Dallas, TX: BenBella Books

Capra, F. (1996). *The Web of Life.* New York: Anchor-Doubleday.

Carrel, A. (1961). *Man the Unknown.* London: Universe Books.

Chaitow, L. and Trenev, N. (1990) *Probiotics.* London: Thorsens.

Colbin, A. (1983) *The Book of Whole Meals.* New York: Ballantine Books.

Colbin, A. (1986). *Food and Healing*. New York: Ballantine Books.

Colbin, A. (1989). *The Natural Gourmet*. New York: Ballantine Books.

Dadd, D. (1986). *The Nontoxic Home*. Los Angeles: Jeremy Tarcher.

De Langre, J. (1990). *Seasalt's Hidden Powers*. Magalia, CA: Happiness Press.

Dune, L. (1990). *Nutrition Almanac*. New York: McGraw Hill.

Esko, E. (1981). *The Cancer Prevention Diet*. Brookline, MA: East West Foundation.

Esko, W. (1980). *Macrobiotic Cooking for Everyone*. Tokyo: Japan Publications.

Estella, M. (1986). *Natural Foods Cookbook*. Tokyo: Japan Publications.

Fallon, S. (1995). *Nourishing Traditions*. San Diego, CA: Promotion Publishing.

France, R. (1982). *Healing Naturally*. Boulder, CO: Amaizeing Books.

Gaeddert, A. (1998). *Healing Digestive Disorders*. Berkeley, CA: N. Atlantic Books.

Gagne, S. (1990). *The Energetics of Food*. Santa Fe, NM: Spiral Science Publishing.

Gates, D. (1996). *The Body Ecology Diet*. Decatur, GA: B.E.D. Publications.

Gittleman, A. (1993). *Guess What Came to Dinner?* Garden City, New York: Avery Publishing Group

Haas, E. (1999). *Detox from damaging habits*. In Nichols, T. & Faass, N., (Ed.).

Optimal Digestion: New Strategies for Achieving Digestive Health. (pp. 262- 271). New York: Avon Books.

Hardy, J. (1996). *Mercury Free*. Gabriel Rose Press. 800-345-0096.

Harper, V. (2002). *Controlling Crohn's Disease The Natural Way*. New York, NY Kensington Publishing Group.

Hawken, P. (1993). *The Ecology of Commerce*. New York: Harper Collins.

Hawken, P. (1999). *Natural Capitalism*. Boston: Little, Brown & Company.

Hillman, J. (1996). *The Soul's Code*. New York: Random House.

Horowitz, R. MD. (2013). *Why Can't I Get Better? Solving the Mystery of Lyme & Chronic Disease*. New York. St. Martin's Press.

Howell, E. (1985). *Enzyme Nutrition*. Wayne, N.J.: Avery Publishing Group.

Hyman, M. MD. (2009). The UltraMind Solution. New York. Scribner.

Illich, I. (1976). *Medical Nemesis*. New York: Pantheon Books.

Jack, A. (1996). *Amber Waves Of Grain*. New York: Random House.

Jensen, B. (1981). *Tissue Cleansing Through Bowel Management*. Escondido, CA: B.J.E. Publishing.

Jensen, B. (1984). *Doctor-Patient Handbook*. Escondido, CA: B.J.E. Publishing.

Jensen, B. (1990). *Empty Harvest*. New York: Avery Publishing Group.

Korngold, E. (1999). *Chinese Medicine and Digestion*. Nichols, T. & Faass, N., (Ed.) *Optimal Digestion: New Strategies for Achieving Digestive Health*. (pp.384-402). New York: Avon Books.

Kotzsch, R. (1985). *Macrobiotics Yesterday and Today*. Tokyo: Japan Publications.

Kripalu Center for Holistic Health, (1984). *The Self Health Guide*. Lenox, MA: Kripalu Publications.

Kulvinskas, V. (1994) *Don't Dine Without Enzymes*. Hot Springs, AR: Love Foods Inc.

Kulvinskas, V. (1986) *Survival In The 21st Century*. London: UBIK Media.

Kushi, A. (1985). *The Changing Seasons Macrobiotic Cookbook*. Wayne, N.J.: Avery Publishing Group.

Kushi, M. (1977). *The Book of Macrobiotics*. Tokyo: Japan Publications.

Kushi, M. (1978). *Natural Healing Through Macrobiotics*. Tokyo: Japan Publications.

Kushi, M. (1980). *How to See Your Health: The Book of Visual Diagnosis*. Tokyo: Japan Publications.

Kushi, M. (1983). *The Cancer Prevention Diet*. New York: St. Martin's Press.

Lambert, B. (2010). A Compromised Generation. Boulder, CO. Sentient Publications.

Lappe, F. (1971). *Diet For A Small Planet*. New York: Ballantine Books.

Lipski, E. (2012). *Digestive Wellness*. New York. McGraw-Hill

Mader, S. (1997). *Inquiry Into Life*. Dubuque, IA: Wm. C. Brown Publishers.

Meade, M. (1993). *Men And The Water Of Life.* San Francisco: Harper Collins.

Miller, G. (2000). *Living in the Environment.* Boston: Brooks Cole Publishing.

Miller, S. (1979). *Food for Thought.* Englewood Cliffs, N.J.: Prentice Hall.

Monte, T. (1993). *World Medicine.* New York: Tarcher Putnam.

Monte, T. (2005). *Unexpected Recoveries.* New York: St. Martin's Press.

Moore, T. (1996). *The Education of the Heart.* New York: Harper Collins.

Moyers, B. (1993). *Healing and The Mind.* New York: Doubleday.

Mullin, G. MD. (2011). *The Inside Tract: Your Good Gut Guide to Great Digestive Health.* New York. Rodale.

Murry, M. (1993). *The Healing Power of Foods.* Rocklin, CA: Prima Publishing.

Myss, C. (1996). *Anatomy of the Spirit.* New York: Harmony Books.

Naidu, A.S. (2013). *Redox Life.* Pomona, CA. Bio-Rep Media.

Nichols, T. & Faass, N., editors (1999). *Optimal Digestion: New Strategies for Achieving Digestive Health.* New York: Avon Books.

Null, G. (1994). *The 90's Healthy Body Book.* Deerfield Beach, FL: Health Communications Inc.

Ohlgren, S. (2002). *Cellular Cleansing Made Easy.* Longmont, CO: Genetic Press.

Ohlren, S. (2006). *The 28-Day Cleansing Program.* Longmont, CO: Genetic Press.

Ohsawa, G. (1965). *Zen Macrobiotics.* Los Angeles: Ohsawa Foundation.

Ornstein, D. (1976). *Medicine Today, Healing Tomorrow.* Millbrae, CA: Celestial Arts

Pimentel, M. (2006). *A New IBS Solution.* Sherman Oaks, CA: Health Point Press.

Price, W. (1938). *Diet and Physical Degeneration.* Los Angeles: Keats Publishing.

Pitchford, P. (1993). *Healing With Whole Foods.* Berkeley, CA: North Atlantic Books.

Plummer, N. (1999). Friendly flora. In Nichols, T. & Faass, N., (Ed.). *Optimal Digestion: New Strategies for Achieving Digestive Health.*

(pp. 46-54). New York: Avon Books.

Robbins, J. (1987). *Diet for a New America.* Walpole, N.H.: Stillpoint Publishing.

Robbins, J. (1996). *Reclaiming Our Health.* Tiburon, CA: H.J. Kramer Inc.

Robbins, J. (2001). *The Food Revolution.* Berkeley, CA: Conari Press.

Robbins, O. (1994). *Choices For Our Future.* Summertown, TN: Book Publishing. (With Sol Solomon.)

Rosenbaum, M. (1999). *Immunity against invaders.* In Nichols, T. & Faass, N., (Ed.). *Optimal Digestion: New Strategies for Achieving Digestive Health.* (pp.35-46). New York: Avon Books.

Santillo, H. (1991). *Food Enzymes.* Prescott, AZ: Hohm Press.

Saputo, L. (1999). *Harmful flora.* In Nichols, T. & Faass, N., (Ed.). *Optimal Digestion: New Strategies for Achieving Digestive Health.* (pp. 54-62). New York: Avon Books.

Saputo, L. & Faass, N. (2002). *Boosting Immunity.* Novato, CA: New World Library.

Sattilaro, A. (1984). *Recalled by Life.* Boston: Houghton Mifflin.

Scala, J. (2000). *Eating Right for a Bad Gut.* New York: Penguin Books

Schulze, R. (1999). *There Are No Incurable Diseases.* Santa Monica, CA: Natural Healing Publications.

Schulze, R. (2003). *Healing Colon Disease Naturally.* Santa Monica, CA: Natural Healing Publications.

Sears, B. (1995). *The Zone.* New York: Harper Collins.

Sehnert, K. (1989). *The Garden Within.* Burlingame, CA: World Health Publishers.

Serinus, J. (1986). *Psychoimmunity and the Healing Process.* Berkeley, CA: Celestial Arts.

Stanchich, L. (1989). *Power Eating Program.* Asheville, NC: Healthy Products.

Thompson, L. (1999). *Our Children Are What Our Children Eat.* San Diego, CA: Dr. Laura Thompson Press.

Trenev, N. (1999). *Probiotics: Nature's Internal Healers.* New York: Avery Publishing

Van Cauwenberghe, M. (1985). *Macrobiotic Home Remedies.* Tokyo: Japan Publications.

Waxman, D. (2002). *The Great Life Handbook.* Philadelphia, PA: DWE, LLC.

Weil, A. (1988). *Health and Healing.* Boston: Houghton Mifflin.

Weil, A. (1990). *Natural Health, Natural Medicine.* Boston: Houghton Mifflin.

Acknowledgements

First of all to my parents, Dante and Elizabeth Mariani whose love and support and endless encouragement have nourished me my whole life and who taught me by their example how to look for the best in others. To my grandparents, Francis and Julia Mariani and William and Katharine Fulton, whose longevity and connections to the old country inspired me to seek the wisdom of the ancestors and all traditional cultures.

To my wife Megan Moore, for her patience with me, and her creativity and love; and for her passionate myth-making and storytelling. You and I together are one of the things that nourishes me best. As the river gives itself into the ocean...

To our sons Brian Lucas Mariani and Evan Julian Cyrus Mariani. Thank you for your love of stories, your passion for sports and your acceptance of the work that I do. You inspire me. I love you and am so proud of you both.

To all my aunts and uncles living and deceased and to all my first, second and third cousins too numerous to mention...so many family gatherings over all these years!

To my sister Audrey, and to my brothers Christopher and William. I love you. To my many brothers and sisters in-law, and to all my nieces and nephews, inlaws and outlaws in the United States and in Canada. What an amazing family!

To all my clients and fellow students over all these years whose open inquisitive minds, compassionate hearts, and often suffering bodies motivated and inspired my quest for practical dietary and lifestyle practices that have found fruition in this book.

To friends and family members who have passed away due to cancer or other degenerative diseases. Your memories bless me, your suffering haunts me, and your life on this earth will always inspire and motivate me. I love and miss you all: Nancy Fulton, Ruth Nielsen, Elizabeth Wilkins, Louis Lowenthal, Francis Mariani, William Fulton, Katharine Fulton, Janet Page, Lucinda Hobart, Jadwiga Slanina and many, many others.

Last but not least I want to express my profound gratitude and appreciation for The Great Spirit that moves through all things; for this magnificent planet earth, for the miracle of health and the vital mysteries of the human body.

"This we know. The earth does not belong to man; man belongs to the earth. This we know. All things are connected like the blood which unites us all in one family. Will you teach your children what we have taught our children? That the earth is our mother? Whatever befalls the earth befalls the sons of the earth. Man did not weave the web of life, he is merely a strand within it. Whatever he does to the web, he does to himself."

These words, for many years were attributed to Chief Seattle, (Sealth) who was the leader of the Duwanish Tribe in the Washington Territory; in a letter to then US President Franklin Pierce in 1854 to mark the transfer of ancestral Indian Lands to the US Government. More recently they have been attributed to poet Ted Perry.

Section 4 - What's Next

What Lies Ahead?

When I look back over the forty years that have passed since I first started learning about the connections between nutrition education and health, two qualities come to mind; *persistence* and *belief*. Early in my quest I developed the strong belief that health and disease *were not* accidents *of* nature but the direct result of a more or less cooperative relationship *with* nature. I had a strong belief that the biological/ecological principles in evidence in the world *around us* could have and would have a direct bearing on the ebb and flow of life and health and well-being, *within us*.

Persistence in these beliefs forced me to prove to myself their validity and usefulness. How useful these beliefs are will be determined by the readers of this book.

The key to making these connections more apparent and accessible to people everywhere is a better system of health education and a much longer list of passionate and committed health educators. I am one of these health educators as change-agents in the culture at large today. I invite you to take up the vocation if it resonates within you. My persistence in this belief about the pivotal role that health practitioners and health educators play in creating a better health-care system for all is what motivated me to complete the writing of this book. I have a clear vision of what lies ahead of us.

What lies ahead is a *paradigm shift* of epic proportion and significance.

No longer can our society afford to persist in its belief in a magic pharmaceutical bullet, or surgical procedure for *all* the many ills that plague us. At last we are at a point where the medical and economic imperatives point directly at each one of us to become more proactive in our own self-care. The current disease-care system is not sustainable. The current disease-care system is broken beyond the hope of effective repair. We need a new approach.

The principles and practices that I have described in *Healing Digestive Illness* are representative of the kinds of things that will prove to be foundational in the health-care system of the future. To establish this new health-care system will require a new set of beliefs and enormous patience and persistence. As a result we will prevent the suffering of millions and lay the groundwork for global cooperation, economic justice and peace. In this not too distant future time, defined by new principles, priorities and practices, we will re-discover our passion for the stewardship of the earth and each other and move forward in our endless perennial quest for the realization of our full human potentials.

What lies behind us and what lies before us are small matters compared to what lies within us.
Ralph Waldo Emerson

Faith is a Magic

Faith is a magic, small but strong.
It eddies near the edge of Fate,
That vast current that flows along
In whorling fortunes, never straight!
Unstoppable as Fate may be,
It sometimes senses faith's small charm
Aswirl at its periphery
And for its use breaks off some harm
That otherwise stood in our way.

Odds Bodkin
www.oddsbodkin.com

Section 4 - What's Next

The Last Word

To me optimum health is most perfectly defined as *the ability to digest everything!* Food, water, air, people, places, things, conversations, ideas, experiences. Everything. Thank you for reading my book. I wish you health and happiness and *inner abdominal tranquility*...today and in all the days ahead.

Russell Mariani

CPSIA information can be obtained
at www.ICGtesting.com
Printed in the USA
FSOW01n2058040217
30305FS